LAST CALL

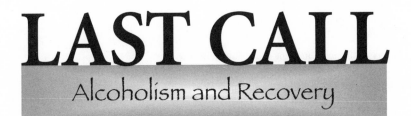

LAST CALL
Alcoholism and Recovery

JACK H. HEDBLOM, M.S.W., PH.D.

Foreword by

PAUL R. MCHUGH, M.D.

2/09
THE JOHNS HOPKINS UNIVERSITY PRESS

Baltimore

© 2007 The Johns Hopkins University Press
All rights reserved. Published 2007
Printed in the United States of America on acid-free paper

9 8 7 6 5 4 3 2 1

The Johns Hopkins University Press
2715 North Charles Street
Baltimore, Maryland 21218-4363
www.press.jhu.edu

Library of Congress Cataloging-in-Publication Data
Hedblom, Jack H., 1938–
    Last call : alcoholism and recovery / Jack H. Hedblom.
        p. ; cm.
    Includes bibliographical references and index.
    ISBN-13: 978-0-8018-8677-5 (hardcover : alk. paper)
    ISBN-13: 978-0-8018-8678-2 (pbk. : alk. paper)
    ISBN-10: 0-8018-8677-5 (hardcover : alk. paper)
    ISBN-10: 0-8018-8678-3 (pbk. : alk. paper)
    1. Alcoholism.   2. Alcoholism—Treatment.   I. Title.
    [DNLM: 1. Alcoholics Anonymous.   2. Alcoholism—therapy.   3. Alcoholism—
psychology. WM 274 H452L 2007]
    RC565.H4389 2007
    616.86'1—dc22

                                                                    2006103534

A catalog record for this book is available from the British Library.

*Special discounts are available for bulk purchases of this book. For more information, please contact
Special Sales at 410-516-6936 or specialsales@press.jhu.edu.*

The Johns Hopkins University Press uses environmentally friendly book materials, including
recycled text paper that is composed of at least 30 percent post-consumer waste, whenever
possible. All of our book papers are acid-free, and our jackets and covers are printed on paper
with recycled content.

For Janice, the perfect partner

AND FOR ALCOHOLICS AND FAMILIES EVERYWHERE

WHO STRUGGLE AGAINST THE TYRANNY OF ADDICTION

Contents

Foreword, by Paul R. McHugh, M.D.   ix

Preface   xiii

1. ALCOHOLICS ANONYMOUS   1

2. A MATTER OF DEFINITION   25

3. ALCOHOL AND THE ALCOHOLIC   45

4. GETTING SOBER   70

5. MENDING:
THE STEPS IN GETTING WELL   87

6. THE COMPONENTS OF SOBRIETY   125

7. THE ALCOHOLIC AND THE FAMILY   148

8. THE ROAD TO A LIFE WELL LIVED:
THE PROMISES   176

Appendix A. Events in the History of Alcoholics Anonymous   189

Appendix B. How It Works, the Steps, and the Traditions   193

Notes   197

References   201

Index   203

Foreword

As everyone who tries quickly learns, the treatment of the alcoholic patient is fraught with frustrations, especially if approached as though, as with other human disorders, one need but point out what reason suggests. The patients have heard all the reasons why they shouldn't drink. Those reasons did not suffice when they heard them from others, and they are not made sufficient by casting them in the language of psychology or calling on the authority of organized medicine or psychiatry for support.

Many therapists, sensing their inadequacy with what is a persistent and devastating behavioral disorder, turn away from these patients figuratively if not literally (as others among the family and friends have), leaving them to struggle on their own. If recovery does occur, it is more by luck than by clinical management. Certainly psychiatrists cannot point to a knowledge base in their discipline as a source of either information or skills on which to build programs of treatment that they or their patients can salute. And why not?

Alcohol abuse and dependency have everything to do with matters of will and agency—issues of mind rather than body. For all that scientists have lately become aware of how alcohol affects neurobiological and psychopharmacological mechanisms, at some crucial level of mind itself—sometimes obviously at the level of pleasure & personal autonomy, sometimes just as obviously at the level of fear and frustration, and always at the level of habit and inclination— the choice to drink alcohol overwhelms everything—duty, meaning, promises, and health—to carry the person along in the slavery of dependence.

One fact has been learned by all therapists who have through repetitive struggles and many frustrations seen the occasional and unexpected success. Only a program led with enthusiasm by a confident leader and structured around confronting and correcting attitudes and assumptions alcoholic patients carry has any chance of succeeding. These programs are hard to find and harder still to copy.

It's as though, to prevail and overcome the conflict of will that flares up to defeat most efforts to change habits or dependence, the patient needs to be faced by a scarred warrior with much experience (hence the scars) for whom the conflict acts to inspire rather than discourage. Must it be that we less-gifted (and less-scarred) therapists can never learn some of the concepts and methods of treatment that these warriors employ and must ever surrender our patients to them for treatment, learning little or nothing in the process? Dr. Hedblom—one of those warriors—sees such an outcome as a failure of the promise of citizenry in the broad community of therapists to teach each other what has come to some either through special gift or through hard experience. Hence, he has written this book.

What it provides—within the organized structure of twelve-step reasoning derived from long experience with and knowledge of Alcoholics Anonymous teaching and practice—is a conceptual grasp of the problem of alcoholism combined with a naturally infectious enthusiasm for treatment that comes with that mastering grasp. Everyone who reads this book (whether therapist, patient, or despairing family member) can draw from both its precepts and its spirit modes of thought and means of action that, employed as suggested, will improve outcomes and provide ways of helping patients in their recovery.

This is not to claim that the path is easy or the treatments simple to apply. Rather, as the author here relates, there are many reasons to expect the kinds of trouble that lead so many to despair—therapists, families, and patients themselves. After all, what could be more demanding for a patient than giving up a behavior that both one's nature and aspects of nurture lead one to enjoy? Such a person needs a steady, step-wise program, coherent in its various stages but ever informed by a vision of what human freedom really is, what helps a slave to alcohol achieve it, and what sustains the commitment of a patient through the arduous process of recovery.

In this sense, this book is a great adventure story told vividly by one who has lived the adventure with many who lost their way with alcohol. Their individual stories, the pitfalls where they stumbled along the twelve-step path, and the humane, psychologically informed efforts and enterprises used successfully to rescue them provide rich instructive detail and bring vividness to the whole narrative.

But the sources of hope and the means for sustaining it are discerned and usefully described here. From that discernment, therapists can take not only a measure of confidence in the possibility of recovery for patients but also much practical advice for developing plans and programs to address this

most daunting clinical problem. And, what I believe might be just as important and valuable about this book, its stories can bring hope to patients and
families. Reasons for optimism in the face of a dread disorder is what they
seek and certainly what they need.

PAUL R. McHUGH, M.D.
Henry Phipps Professor of Psychiatry Emeritus
former Director, Department of Psychiatry and Behavioral Sciences
Johns Hopkins University School of Medicine

Preface

The message of this book is that the disease of alcoholism can be arrested. The alcoholic can get sober and stay that way. A family can understand and make peace with the chaos generated by an alcoholic member. They can learn to adjust to the new family system generated by the recovering sober family member.

Alcoholism is a disease of denial. Paradoxically, its treatment demands self-diagnosis, or at least being able to accept a symptom-generated diagnosis offered by a professional or others affected by the individual's condition. Few diseases are as pervasive as alcoholism. Its devastation includes individual and family systems. Its treatment requires a program as comprehensive as the disease. Everyone close to the alcoholic is affected by his or her drinking. In most cases, the progression of the disease is so slow and subtle that it goes unnoticed until highlighted by a crisis. Its impact is cumulative, however. Lives can be riddled with troubles, personal and social, all related to alcohol, without the connection being understood. The drinker frequently reports that he drinks because he has so many troubles; the truth is that he has so many troubles because he drinks.

This book is about alcoholics and their families. Its focus is on recovery in a Twelve-Step program. Families of alcoholics will learn about the nature of the disease, its treatment, and the role of the family in that treatment. Some sources of family support and treatment are also referenced.

Although there may be other means by which sobriety can be achieved, the program of Alcoholics Anonymous (AA) is the most comprehensive today. Its effectiveness is attested to by the extent of twelve-step facilitation in addiction treatment centers nationwide. No other program has its universal appeal or such a broad range of services. Moreover, its services are free. Alcoholics Anonymous is unique in its insistence that alcoholism is not a symptom of underlying physical or psychological pathology; rather, it defines alcohol as the wellspring of pathologies. Its program focuses on practical living, offering a pragmatic philosophy and a nonreligiously defined spirituality, and it addresses the three aspects of alcoholism: spiritual, physical, and mental.

Most professional treatment programs are compatible with the Alcoholics Anonymous philosophy. In fact, most are strengthened by the inclusion of AA meetings. It provides focus and direction in therapy.

Throughout the ensuing chapters, I include the stories and experiences of alcoholics drawn from sources throughout the country. The stories and anecdotes are all composites, as are the characters telling the stories and the other characters in them. They are abstractions—"ideal types"—and do not reflect the experience or views of any one individual, nor are they intended to represent the position of Alcoholics Anonymous. I use the first-person form of narrative to strengthen the image of specific individual experiences and to convey a feeling of what goes on at an AA meeting.

Many books have been written about Alcoholics Anonymous. Some of these have recounted its history and origins, some have analyzed its programs, and others have attempted to recast it to fit a current fashion in theory or therapy. It is not my intention to recast, add to, or detract from it. Instead, I discuss the AA program with regard to the threefold nature of the disease of alcoholism and let my characters speak for themselves. For better or worse, Alcoholics Anonymous is a program of action accomplished by the afflicted. The membership shares its experience, strength, and hope to facilitate healing. It does not lecture newcomers into sobriety. For this reason, my discussion focuses on the nature of the alcoholic and the practical, day-to-day disciplines that generate sobriety.

LAST CALL

1

ALCOHOLICS ANONYMOUS

The room is small and painted white. It is in the basement of a church named after two saints. Those who attend meetings here regularly call it Two Guys. People have been filing in since 8 p.m., ready for a meeting to begin at 8:30. There is a murmur of conversation and laughter. Coffee and cookies are passed around. As the meeting is opened, attention focuses on a tall, middle-aged man sitting at a table in the front of the room. "My name is Gary, and I'm an alcoholic."

Meetings all over the world begin in the same way: a statement of purpose is read, followed by the Twelve Steps and a declaration of principles, and the introduction of the meeting chairman, who begins with his self-declaration as an alcoholic. Gary's story continues.

"I began drinking in high school. Everyone I knew drank beer at parties and get-togethers. Fake IDs were circulated. I had one that said I was twenty-six years old, and it worked every time. The most popular guy in school altered ID cards. He magnified the last two numbers in the birth date and had a way of picking out individual grains of ink to change the date. He owned a typewriter that matched the type used on the federal draft cards. To top it off, he could put the gloss back on the paper of the card when he finished. A real artist. It cost ten dollars and was a major investment in the '50s.

"What I'm saying is that lots of us drank. Booze was good to me when I started to drink. It did just what it was supposed to do, although at the time, I didn't analyze why I drank, I just liked it. With a little beer in me, I was relaxed around girls. I thought beer made me a better dancer and a better driver. For some reason, I bragged about how much I drank and how often. I wanted a reputation for being a little wild. After a while, I started to believe the stories I told myself. The truth was, like a lot of other kids around me, I was

unsure of myself and more than a little shy. I was a C student with a lot of inner turmoil. It got in the way of adjusting to high school and doing better. It
was caused by my drinking but I didn't know that then. Whatever feelings or
problems I had, I certainly didn't connect them with beer. As a matter of fact,
a friend of mine and I used to ride around on weekend nights drinking beer
and listening to the local rhythm-and-blues station. We didn't get drunk or
even high; we just drank some beer and listened to the blues. I think the show
was called *Jam with Sam*. Like all kids, I was uncertain about myself. Looking
back on those times, I think I was already depending on alcohol for a lot of
things. The important thing was that I didn't think of a good time without
thinking about booze."

As Gary speaks, the audience is quiet and attentive. There are no interrup-
tions. Questions will come later.

"When I graduated from high school, I went into the army. I wanted to get
it over with. I was away from home for the first time. After basic training we
had a big party. I really got drunk. Everyone drank a lot. The army was a
three-year drunk during which I learned photography. I had a talent for photography. That's what I do today. I found out that I could drink more than
anyone around me. I was the guy who drove everyone home. I didn't have
hangovers or get into trouble. I didn't drink for any reason; I just drank. I
know now that people around me thought of me as a boozer. When I was invited to a party, people bought extra booze. I came early and stayed late.

"After the army, I started taking pictures, mostly of children. Because I
worked for myself, I drank when I felt like it. At first it was just the regular
times when others were drinking. Later I drank all the time; I got good at taking baby pictures in my home. I would set up a background and stuff and use
an excuse to get the mother out of the room. 'May I have a glass of water?' As
soon as she left the room, I would reach over and pinch the hell out of a toe or
whatever I could reach. As the baby opened up to scream, I would snap the
picture. If I was quick the tears rushing to the eyes would give me a good
sparkle and the open mouth looked like a big smile. So help me, the pictures
looked great. If you missed the first one, however, it was over for the day. The
mother would come back into the room with my water and the job would be
over. I didn't really hurt the babies, but I sure got their attention. Needless to
say, this technique didn't work with verbal children. I opened a studio and
expanded my business to include school portraits and advertising. My business flourished and my drinking flourished along with it."

Gary does not lecture or underline parts of his story. He does not teach. The lesson is in the story and its relevance to the audience.

"Along the way, I picked up a wife and child. They insisted I spend time with them. I ran from responsibility and fought with her. I spent all of my time at the studio or at the bar. I had hired a manager and another photographer, and I did less and less work myself. I could have written the book on how to lose a business. Fran and I separated when I got my second DWI. I hardly knew myself. Another ten months went by. I was postponing the court appearance on the DWI for as long as I could. I was never really drunk, but I was never really sober. I guess I was just saturated. Things came and went, and I didn't seem to care. I was tired all the time. My stomach seemed to be in a constant state of upset. My hands shook in the morning until I had a few 'jolts.' Whole pieces of time seemed to disappear.

"One day at the studio, while I was sitting in my office drinking, the police came to arrest me. A few days before, I had evidently hit another car, injured a passenger, and fled. A witness had written down my license plate number. I was taken in handcuffs to the police station. When I was in lockup waiting for a bondsman, I went into withdrawal and had a seizure. I woke up in the hospital in a locked section of the alcohol ward. Three days had gone by; I almost died. When I felt up to it two weeks later, I protested to my doctor that I didn't belong there. In the midst of death, I was frightened of being called an alcoholic. My troubles were inconveniences. My real fear was that I would have to stop drinking.

"I was in the hospital for a month and in a therapy program for another thirty days. The doctor told me with absolute certainty that if I drank again, I would die. My liver was enlarged. I was still yellow. I didn't think I could live without booze. The state helped me. I was sentenced to a year in the county jail and two years probation. I served my first six months hard time and my last six months on work release. In jail I attended AA meetings and they were a part of my probation. I don't think I could have made it without the jail time. I don't recommend it for everybody but it worked for me.

"The rest of my story is a success. Fran and I are back together, and I work for a large studio. Maybe I'll open another studio, I don't know. I live one day at a time, and right now I'm concentrating on keeping my life simple and meaningful to me and my family. I'm off probation and sponsor other people trying to get sober. I'm a regular speaker at the jail AA meetings. I don't lecture on the evils of booze or what's wrong with everybody else. I just talk about what happened to me. I'm grateful that a lot more didn't happen to me. The woman I hurt in the accident recovered. I'm in one piece and so is my family. A lot of others aren't so lucky.

"You know, when I went to my first meeting right after the hospital, a guy came up to me and asked if I felt as bad as I looked. That pissed me off, but I didn't say anything. He kept right on, hoping that I felt bad for a long time and further hoped that I would remember it. I'll never forget what he said next (just when I was going to tell him where to put the meeting table); 'You don't have to live through this again.' He was right. I haven't had to. I didn't thank him then but I should have. My subject tonight is 'Powerless over Alcohol.' Let's open the meeting for discussion."

What you have just read is an introduction to sharing at an Alcoholics Anonymous meeting. It is called a "drunk-a-logue." It is the sharing of experience and hope with other alcoholics. It is an affirmation of sobriety. When Gary shares his story about the way he arrested his disease, he points the way to recovery for the alcoholic who still drinks or the newcomer who wants desperately to get well. Paradoxically, it is in this way that Gary himself remains sober.

As an organization, Alcoholics Anonymous grew out of the need of two desperate men to get sober and a serendipitous meeting. It is hard to believe that the present organization and its worldwide membership of millions has evolved in a little more than fifty years. Even more incredible is the fact that this growth has occurred with almost no advertising, a decentralized authority and organization, and a rigidly maintained posture of nonownership and poverty. It may be that AA has grown in proportion to the need for what it offers. Its history will help us understand the content of AA as it exists today. It has changed over time yet remains entirely consistent with the vision of its founders.

The Foundations of AA

The chain of events that created Alcoholics Anonymous began when one of its cofounders, Bill Wilson, was visited by an old drinking buddy, Ebby T., who had stopped drinking with the help of a nondenominational religious organization called the Oxford Group. Founded by Frank Buchman in 1921, the group was spiritual in nature and intended to recapture the essence of first-century Christianity. The members of the Oxford Group, or, as it was called after 1939, the Moral Re-Armament Group, emphasized prayer and the importance of seeking God's guidance in all matters. They relied on studying the scriptures for guidance and in turn developed their own literature.

Members of the Oxford Group sought to achieve spiritual regeneration by surrendering to God through rigorous self-examination, confessing their character defects to another human being, making restitution for harm done to others, and giving without thought of reward. They did, however, accept contributions.[1] Morally, the group relied on what they called their four absolutes:

1. Absolute honesty
2. Absolute purity
3. Absolute unselfishness
4. Absolute love

Additionally, they advocated what they referred to as the five Cs and the five procedures. The Cs were:

1. Confidence
2. Confession
3. Conviction
4. Conversion
5. Continuance

The procedures were a bit more complicated:

1. Give in to God
2. Listen to God's directions
3. Check guidance
4. Restitution
5. Sharing for witness and confession[2]

With this set of mandates in mind, Oxford Group members attempted to influence community leaders and to motivate others to perform good works. They viewed themselves as modern apostles, patterned after the original twelve. Drawing from the general public, they wanted to create generations of apostles devoted to solving existing social problems through living by and extolling Christian virtues. Their concern with social and individual problems (salvation) attracted alcoholics to the movement. The group relied heavily on publicity generated by converting prominent people to the movement. They began neighborhood groups, much as AA was to do later.

The meetings were concerned with the process of leading the moral life and team guidance of the lives of its members. In many ways, the meetings were similar to AA meetings of today. The principal difference, however, was that the Oxford Group meetings tended to be pushy and authoritarian, whereas AA meetings were more indirect. In AA, individuals were led to revelation rather than pushed to it. Alcoholics seemed to resist the push. They viewed their problems as personal, not global. They needed to save themselves to get sober. Like early AA meetings, Oxford Group meetings were held in the homes of members. Those things that separated the alcoholics from the Oxford Group members were the great differences in their intentions. The alcoholics may have wanted to save the world, but first they wanted to save themselves. Oxford Group members could afford to be more general in their concerns.

As alcoholics became more involved with the Oxford Group movement, the movement seemed to move further away from them. Dr. Bob (a cofounder of AA) was a member of an Oxford Group for three years, during which time he said his spiritual search began. His drinking continued.

The Oxford Group's influence on AA was to be significant, with its "absolutes," its "C's," and its traditions providing inspiration for many of the Steps and Traditions in Alcoholics Anonymous. AA, however, was not to have the Oxford Group's emphasis on community prayer, reliance on Christian dogma, or its need for publicity.

Bill Wilson's friend Ebby T. had tried to get sober over and over, but with no success. When Ebby finally did achieve a period of sobriety in the Oxford Group, he attributed it to a religious experience and commitment. Wilson did not rush to conversion. He was, however, haunted by his friend's epiphany and subsequent sobriety. Bill would undergo a number of conversions of his own. He began to think of alcoholism as a disease, not unlike cancer. He recognized the panacea (abstinence), yet he knew he was powerless over his dependence on alcohol. "For several days I went on drinking. But in no waking hour was the thought of my friend absent from my mind. I could not forget what he said."[3] In the kinship of common suffering, one alcoholic had been talking to another. Bill was admitted to his last detox at Towns Hospital on December 11, 1934, under the care of Dr. William Silkworth.

In the hospital, Bill was visited by his friend Ebby, who described the Oxford Group's approach to abstinence. Bill was still resistant to any inclusion of God in a formula for getting well. He asked Ebby what his secret for sobriety was. Ebby replied, "You admit you are licked; you get yourself honest with yourself; you talk it out with somebody else; you make restitution to the people you have harmed; you try to give of yourself without stint, with no demand for reward; and you pray to whatever God you think there is, even as an experiment."[4]

Bill remained depressed. As his depression deepened, Bill described his feeling as "if the last vestige of my proud obstinacy was crushed. All at once I found myself crying out, 'If there is a God, let him show himself, I am ready to do anything.'"[5] At this point Bill underwent what he later described as a religious spiritual experience. He described himself as feeling ecstasy and described himself as being in another world of consciousness. Whether it was a hallucination or a dream, the experience was to provide impetus for the pursuit of sobriety with no holds barred. The experience of ego deflation at depth, the spiritual experience coupled with the fact of one alcoholic working with another, seemed to have made the circle complete.

As soon as he was discharged from the hospital, he associated himself with the Oxford Group. He wanted to work with drunks. But members of the group were not all enthusiastic about this special focus, and Bill did not get anyone sober.

Bob and Bill Meet

In 1935 Bill Wilson went to Akron, Ohio, on business. Disappointed in his business affairs, he found himself in a hotel, with money in his pocket and the idea in his mind that he was going to get drunk. He recalled that when he tried to help others get sober, he had stayed sober himself. After a series of telephone calls seeking out alcoholics connected with the Oxford Group, he contacted a woman, Henrietta Sieberling, who was "a devout member of the Oxford Group. She invited Bill to her home and arranged a meeting between Bill and Dr. Bob Smith. Dr. Bob, as he was later known, was a 'project' of Mrs. Sieberling's, who was a close friend of Smith's wife. Bob Smith was a chronic alcoholic and a drug-dependent surgeon with a failing practice; he had no hope of reversing his decline. Reluctantly, Bob Smith met with Bill Wilson in the Sieberling home."[6]

After Ebby visited him in the hospital, Bill had begun reading the works of William James. He identified three common denominators in all of the clinical cases that James reported. "These insights became important to Bill in his thinking about the plight of the alcoholic and his need for spiritual help. (He would later say that James, though long in his grave, had been a founder of Alcoholics Anonymous.) Of the three common denominators in James's case histories, the first was calamity: each person James described had met utter defeat in some vital area of his life. All human resources had failed to resolve his problems. Each person had been utterly desperate. The next common point was admission of defeat. Each of the individuals acknowledged his own defeat as utter and absolute. The third common denominator was an appeal to a higher power. This cry for help could take many forms or might not be in religious terms."[7]

In the population James described, he reported: "The responses were equally varied. Some had thunderbolt experiences, as did Saint Paul on the road to Damascus; others had slow, gradual transformation experiences. Whatever the type of the experience, however, it brought the sufferer into a new state of consciousness and so opened the way to release from the old problems."[8] Wilson was later to define this in the AA context as a "spiritual awakening."

Dr. Robert Smith was fifty-five years old at the time of his meeting with Bill Wilson. He was fifteen years older than Bill. His drinking had begun when he was a student at Dartmouth College and manifested itself as a problem early in his studies. He all but failed in his studies at Rush Medical College in Chicago.[9] His drinking punctuated his career with failure. At the time of his meeting with Wilson, he had been an active member of the Oxford Group for three years but had continued to drink throughout.

Dr. Bob later said that he could not remember ever feeling much worse than he did on the afternoon he met Bill. He had agreed to the meeting only because he was very fond of Henrietta and Ann had already committed them to going. But he made Ann promise that they would stay only fifteen minutes ... Bill recalled, "After dinner, which he did not eat, Henrietta discreetly put us off in her little library. There Bob and I talked until eleven o'clock."

What caused Dr. Bob to stay for the evening, instead of fleeing, as planned? To begin with, he quickly realized that this Bill Wilson knew what he was talking about. Dr. Bob had read a great deal about alcoholism and had heard the opinion of fellow professionals who had treated alcoholics. But Bill was the first person he had talked with who knew from his own experience what alcoholism was. "In other words, he talked my language," said Bob. "He knew all the answers and not because he picked them up in his readings."

It was not only personal experience that Bill shared that day. In addition to the influence of William James, a vital part of his message was the medical view that Dr. Silkworth had explained and had urged him to present to prospective "converts." It is ironic that Bob, a physician, should learn about alcoholism as an illness from Bill, a stockbroker; however, Dr. Bob's medical training may have helped him grasp what was then a radical concept.

While Bill Wilson and Dr. Bob Smith hit it off from the very first talk at Henrietta's home, neither had any way of anticipating the monumental ramifications that would ensue from that encounter.[10]

Whether by coincidence or by chemistry, these two alcoholics began the work that would dominate the rest of their lives; they based their sobriety on working with other alcoholics within a moral and ethical framework, an amalgam of philosophy, religion, and the experiences of alcoholics getting sober.

The Emergence of Alcoholics Anonymous

Bob and Bill and others continued to work with the Oxford Group. The alcoholics focused more and more on helping other drunks, while the other group members were more cosmopolitan in their intentions. The alcoholic contingent found the Oxford Group's aggressive evangelism and team guidance of their lives too authoritarian. The moral absolutes of the movement were important to recovery but needed a new wrapping. A particularly thorny problem was the question of publicity and public identity. Because of the stigma attached to alcoholism, most of the alcoholic members wanted to remain anonymous. They wanted to avoid the failure of a publicly identified member getting drunk and implying the failure of the group. The Oxford Group relied heavily on prominent names as a way of introducing or gaining new members.

The break was imminent. It occurred shortly after the publication of *Alcoholics Anonymous* in 1939. There was a fear that the message of Alcoholics Anonymous and its program would be lost. Yet by 1950, AA membership numbered in the hundreds of thousands.

AA Early Years

The Twelve Traditions of the Alcoholics Anonymous program were forged from experience, out of the need to protect the fledgling truth from contamination. The program was to be decentralized, uninvolved with social or topical issues, politics or religion, unencumbered by property or money, avowedly nonprofessional, self-supporting, nonpromoted, and above all anonymous. AA continues to be nonprofessional; that is, it is not directed in any way by physicians, psychiatrists, social workers, clerics, or any other kind of professionally trained group. Its collective wisdom is derived from the shared experience of its membership. The framework in which that sharing takes place was hammered out of the experience of alcoholics working with other alcoholics toward the goal of long-range sobriety. The Traditions provided an organizational format that has supported the growth of AA worldwide. The ethical and moral foundations of the program were stated with equal pragmatism. Bill Wilson wrote the Steps guided by the influences of the "absolutes" of the Oxford Group, the writings of William James, and the influence of W. D. Silkworth, the first medical friend of AA.

In the early history of AA's split from the Oxford Group, considerable disagreement existed between the eastern and midwestern factions of the newly founded Alcoholics Anonymous. The midwesterners still tended to identify themselves as Oxford members and talked about the Oxford Group's "absolutes." The eastern contingent, on the other hand, increasingly emphasized the disease concept of alcoholism and focused on the individual's obsession with alcohol. "In Akron and vicinity they still talked about the Oxford Group's absolutes . . . This dose was found to be too rich for New Yorkers, and we had abandoned the expressions. But all of us, East and West, were placing emphasis on Dr. Silkworth's expression, describing the alcoholic's dilemma: the obsession plus the allergy. And now we knew from experience that the new prospect had to accept Step 1 or get no place."[11]

Split from the Oxford Group

During its early years, Alcoholics Anonymous continued to identify itself with the Oxford Group. However, the Oxford Group drew unwanted publicity to itself when its founder Buchman was quoted in the newspapers as having said, "I thank heaven for a man like Adolf Hitler who built a front line defense against the anti-Christ of Communism. Think what it would mean to the world if Hitler surrendered to God. Through such a man God could control a nation and solve every problem. Human problems aren't economic, they're moral, and they can't be solved by immoral measures." This was sufficient to label Buchman a "Nazi" in the press. Concomitantly, representative members of the Oxford Group had grown increasingly disapproving of alcoholics focusing on their particular needs within the group's framework. The Oxford Group moved from meeting in small intimate groups to holding large gatherings. "In 1938, after Oxford University requested that the group, because of the controversy, no longer use its name, it took the name Moral Re-armament, abbreviated to MRA. Increasingly, it worked with national and world assemblies. A number of early followers withdrew from the movement dissatisfied with the shift from individual emphasis to mass methods."[12]

Bill Wilson led the split with the Oxford Group while recognizing its contribution to him and to AA. Dr. Bob and other members stayed until 1939. Wilson's reasons for leaving the group were somewhat misunderstood, and he made a number of extensive statements about the situation. He adopted those parts of the Oxford Group's philosophy which he thought best served alcoholics but rejected others. For example, he rejected the principle of aggressive evangelicalism, convinced that its impact was divisive and would not address alcoholics' needs. He rejected the importance of personal publicity or prominence in the work that was to be done. He avoided using the term *absolute* in front of such concepts as honesty, purity, unselfishness, and the like because he believed that absolutes turn people away. He thought that all forms of coercion, direct and indirect, negatively affected work with alcoholics.

The principles of tolerance and love had to be more overtly emphasized in practice than they were in the Oxford Group, particularly tolerance. "We can never say to anyone (or insinuate) that he must agree to our formula or be excommunicated. The atheist may stand up in an AA meeting denying God, yet reporting how he has been helped in other ways. Experience tells us he will presently change his mind, but nobody can tell him he must do so."[13] Wilson continued on this line, suggesting that no religion would be favored over another. In this way, the program could embrace the orthodox, the unorthodox, and the unbeliever as well. Wilson was to find support for this interpretation when his initial effort at codifying the AA program was passed among the membership for modification or approval.

Wilson was largely true to his principles. The organization eschewed money, with the exception of a $5,000 grant from the Rockefeller Foundation, which was placed in an account to be drawn on as needed. This largely went to pay off the mortgage on Bob Smith's home. Bill and Bob continued to administer AA as a roughly defined organization and did so by example. Wilson, in particular, was poverty stricken and yet brought alcoholics into his home and shared his roof with them until they could make it on their own. When Bill was offered a job as a counselor in the very hospital where he had undergone detoxification on four separate occasions, he was forced to turn it down. He felt that accepting it would have been a violation of the principles of AA. His life at this point was completely devoted to AA, and he seemed to have lost all interest in other economic ventures.

At a low point in his financial life, late in 1937, Bill made a trip to Detroit and Cleveland looking for work. He didn't find a job, but he did visit Bob and Ann in Akron. It was on this visit that the two men conducted a formal review of their work of the past two years. What they came to realize as the result of that review was astounding. Bill may have been stretching things when he declared that at least twenty cases had been sober for a couple of years. But by counting everybody who seemed to have found sobriety in New York and Akron, they concluded that more than forty alcoholics were staying dry as a result of the program. "As we carefully rechecked this score it suddenly burst upon us that a new light was shining into the dark world of the alcoholic," Wilson wrote. "A benign chain reaction, one alcoholic carrying the good news to the next, had started outward from Dr. Bob and me. Conceivably it could one day circle the whole world. What a tremendous thing that realization was! At last we were sure. There would be no more flying totally blind. We actually wept for joy, and Bob and Ann and I bowed our heads in silent thanks."[14] Their gratitude would have surprised some. Bill, who turned forty-two that year, was jobless, while Dr. Bob at fifty-eight was in danger of losing his house. But Bill had nearly three years' sobriety; Bob had two and a half years.

The "Big Book" and the Steps

Bill Wilson began writing what was to become the bible of AA, *Alcoholics Anonymous,* colloquially referred to as the "Big Book," in March or April of 1938. Although there was at least one offer of publication, Wilson and the group decided to publish their own book and, in this way, to own it. This began a tradition of AA publishing and controlling its own literature. "Bill wrote the twelve steps while lying in a bed at 182 Clinton St. with pencil in hand and pad of yellow scratch paper on his knee. He wrote them in bed," said Lois, "not because he was really sick, but he wasn't feeling well and if he could lie down he did: he got into bed, that being the best place to think. He completed the first draft of the Twelve Steps in about a half hour, then kept on writing until he felt he should stop and review what he had written. Numbering the Steps, he found they added up to twelve—'A symbolic number,' he thought, because of the twelve apostles, and soon became convinced that the Society should have twelve steps."[15] When *Alcoholics Anonymous* was published in 1939, the first paragraph of the foreword read: "We, of Alcoholics Anonymous, are more than one hundred men and women who have recovered from a seemingly hopeless state of mind and body. To show other alcoholics *precisely how we have recovered* is the main purpose of this book."[16] With the publication of the Big Book and the formulation of the Twelve Steps of AA, the movement was well on its way. (Appendix A lists significant dates in the evolution of the program. The Twelve Steps, Twelve Traditions, and How It Works, read at the beginning of each meeting, are included as Appendix B.)

The history of AA is remarkable for the coincidences surrounding its beginning. Its existence today lends credence to the old bromide that nothing can stop an idea whose time has come. The number of people served by the AA program has increased to millions throughout the world; the organizational structure of AA has evolved to handle its informational and distribution needs. The doctrines of the program have not changed. Although meetings may vary somewhat in format, their content as described in the literature is generally adhered to. What is most incredible about the organization is

the smoothness with which it operates in the face of complete decentralization and its almost fanatical commitment to anarchy.

Meetings

Decentralization is so fundamental to AA's being that each group, regardless
of size, is autonomous and self-supporting. Because its anarchism is flavored
with democracy, it may include virtually everyone who wants to identify
himself or herself as a member: "The only requirement of AA is a desire to
stop drinking." "We finally said to ourselves, 'Who are we to keep anybody
out?'" To many desperate drunks, AA is the court of last appeal. "How can we
slam the door on anybody who stands up . . . We must always take the risk, no
matter who comes in."[17]

The Fourth Tradition of AA says, in short, that each group is autonomous
and self-supporting through its own contributions, except in matters affecting other groups or AA as a whole. This means that an AA group can exercise
its right to be wrong. "Any two or three gathered together for sobriety can call
themselves an AA group provided that as a group they have no other affilia-
tion. This means that these two or three alcoholics could try for sobriety in
any way they like. They can disagree with any or all of AA's principles and still
call themselves an AA group."[18]

All meetings are opened by a reading of the prologue, either a prologue
unique to the region but based on the first page of the chapter of *Alcoholics
Anonymous* or a simple reading of the part of the book called "How It
Works." After the reading of the prologue, a member reads the Steps and the
Traditions out loud. The group secretary, an individual elected by the membership to serve a limited term of office, reads a short bulletin and introduces
the invited speaker for the evening. At a general meeting, the speaker describes himself: he tells how it was when he was drinking, how he got sober,
and how it is today. In this way, he qualifies himself as a member of AA, talks
about the impact of the program on his alcoholism, and then talks about the
impact of the program in the daily conduct of his life. Although such a
"drunk-a-logue" can take as much time as the speaker wishes, it ordinarily
lasts for the first twenty minutes or so of the normal meeting time of one
hour. After the speaker has finished, he suggests a topic and begins to call on
people in the group to "share."

Sharing involves talking about one's self, one's experience, one's strength, and one's hope in terms of staying sober one day at a time. Subjects for discussion are drawn from the Big Book or may focus on a given problem or topic. Although people speak frankly about themselves and their experiences, the meetings are generally not a place for confession. Before speaking, or sharing, people introduce themselves by first name and identify themselves as alcoholics. Getting to know someone in AA occurs on the basis of what is presented. Evaluation of individuals is therefore based on what is immediately known about them in the program, not on any other criteria. The normal touchstones of identity and social class in this culture do not exist in an AA meeting. It is often said that people are willing to share more about themselves and their most private moments in AA meetings than at any other encounter in their lives, and yet they may not know each other's last names. One can know people intimately at AA meetings and never know what they do for a living, what neighborhood they live in, or how much money they have, unless these details are disclosed at a meeting. As clichéd as it sounds, people are evaluated on the basis of what they are rather than what they have or who they are. This is not to suggest that a normal shaking out does not result in the creation of a social hierarchy. As in any other social situation, people with similar interests, backgrounds, or education tend to gravitate to one another, although this is certainly not without variation. Another hierarchy is based on the longevity of sobriety or quality of the individual's program as perceived by others. There are leaders and followers, stars and superstars in AA. There are persons who are known to chair entertaining, "good" meetings, and there are others whose messages are more subdued and perhaps even boring.

Despite these distinctions, the meetings continue at a pace, and it is generally agreed that whatever occurs at a meeting needed to occur. As a matter of fact, one can often hear it said that all meetings are good, some are simply better than others. Some say that if you haven't been to a bad meeting, you haven't been to enough meetings.

Meetings can be formed by any group of people who want to meet once a week to discuss sobriety. The meetings may be of any type and may or may not represent a special interest group. For example, there are women's groups, gay groups, groups exclusively dedicated to the medical profession, the legal profession, and so on. The meetings may take place anywhere that is mutually convenient. Space may be rented in a church or synagogue, or meetings may take place on a revolving basis in people's homes, as was the case in the early years of Alcoholics Anonymous. The meetings may be of many types. They may be open meetings where the public, while not invited, is welcomed. The thought is that people who are curious about AA meetings frequently have a reason for the curiosity, and an open meeting gives them an opportunity to attend without declaring themselves alcoholic. Closed meetings admit only persons who describe themselves as alcoholics and who are attending to treat their disease. Some meetings may be devoted exclusively to the Steps. At such a meeting, one Step a week is considered until all twelve have been considered, then the cycle begins again. All meetings may fit into one of two categories. They can be speaker meetings, where an individual speaks on a given subject for the entire hour, or they can be discussion meetings, where the speaker may take up to twenty minutes and then open a discussion on a subject of his choosing.

Regardless of the type or the place, all meetings have something in common. They begin with a declaration of purpose, a reading of the Twelve Steps involved in sobriety and the Twelve Traditions, and a focus on one aspect of alcoholism or another. They are a community sharing moral and ethical concerns and providing social gatherings where help may be sought and is freely given. For the alcoholic, meetings are a necessary action part of the program. I have never heard a satisfactory explanation of what goes on in AA meetings that makes them so essential to the sobriety of an alcoholic. Perhaps it is the experience of the fellowship. Slips, or returns to alcoholic drinking, however, frequently begin with declining attendance at meetings. It is almost as if the individual in the process of falling away from AA and gradually disassociating himself from the fellowship of meetings undergoes a kind of deconversion. He stops placing his faith in the process of AA as a way of life. He loses faith in the process that got him sober and kept him sober. He either takes his sobriety for granted or begins to believe that he is keeping himself sober. In many ways this is a type of loss of identity. It is as if the individual loses his sense of "fit" in the world. He ceases to surround himself with reminders of his past affirmations of his potential as an alcoholic. In the language of the AA founders, perhaps he has lost the magic that occurs when one alcoholic works with another toward the goal of sobriety. While there is no guarantee that the alcoholic who stops coming to meetings will get drunk, it is certain that he places himself at great risk. This is a life-and-death risk and not to be taken lightly.

The Spirit of Meetings

It is difficult to describe the spirit of the typical AA meeting. The gathering begins about half an hour before the actual start time of the meeting. Everyone seems to be drinking coffee or tea. Often cookies are served. Some people seem to station themselves at the door to greet the newcomers. A general buzz comes from the sound of chairs being set up for the meeting. Literature is put out. Conversations range from everyday chitchat to discussion of the most serious problems. There is a lot of laughter. People look clean and healthy and seem to show a genuine concern for each other.

The meeting is run by its membership, which elects a secretary. The secretary attends a number of other meetings during the week and solicits speakers. It is assumed that all members can chair a meeting equally well and that what occurs at an AA meeting was intended to occur. Somebody arrives early and makes coffee. Some stay after the meeting and clean up. If the people appointed to do these tasks have emergencies and do not show up, others automatically do the work. Voluntary contributions pay for the coffee, cookies, and hall rental, and remaining funds are distributed to state and national AA organizations to support local as well as worldwide information and coordination services.

Above all, meetings are an expression of fellowship. Regardless of the designated type of meeting, they are full of ideas and sayings that address the general process of living. A member shared the following at a newcomers' meeting: "When I came to AA, I knew all about being drunk. I could manage to live every day on the razor's edge—not drunk, not sober, just balanced. I needed the edge to operate normally. If I could manage my alcohol, that is, keep the supply near and feel relaxed about it, no one suspected that I was drinking. They would assume that what they saw was a normal me. It got so that I did not even know what I was really like. I lost myself a while ago. When I hit bottom and sought help, I still wanted it my way. I went to a psychiatrist for about six months. I lied about how much I drank and we chased one therapeutic dragon after another. I invented most of them. He gave me pills and tried to figure out how I got to be crazy. I thought it was the booze that helped me through the day. I drank all through the therapy. After a binge and a car wreck and a depth of despair that I had never known, I called AA and came to a meeting. I gave it up. I had no answers. I knew about living drunk but did not know anything about living sober. I hadn't really been sober for fifteen years. It wasn't enough that I stopped drinking. I had to learn how to live. I had to sort out me from the booze and see what parts of me were real and what part was alcohol. I had to come to grips with my past and learn to live my life to good purpose. I needed to heal.

"People I met at the meeting told me what they had been through. They didn't seem to feel sorry for me but they did tell me that it didn't have to be that way anymore. They also said that if I did what I was told I wouldn't have to go through withdrawal ever again. A lot of what they told me I didn't remember. I was pretty well out of it. I did remember ninety meetings in ninety days. And someone was telling me to do it one day at a time. For a while the slogans and epigrams drove me crazy. They seemed so trite and obvious; they have since come to mean a great deal to me. 'Bring the body and the mind will follow'; for a while that's all I had to bring. Then I began to sense that the program of sobriety at AA was so simple and yet so profound that I just might miss it. A miracle happened. Ninety-one days had passed, and for the first time in years I had not had a drink. I wasn't sure how it happened or for that matter that I had intended it, but it happened. I was sober and scared to death. If I lost my way in this, I would have absolutely nothing.

"The key, somehow or other, was the meetings. I didn't say anything. When I was called on to share, I passed. I did give my first name and admitted I was an alcoholic. Whenever I went to a meeting, I felt better. I identified with some of the stories I heard. Mostly I think I kept coming back because I saw lots of people at the meetings who were sober and happy. It was what the literature said, 'If you want what we have and are willing to go to any lengths to get it'; I wanted what these people had and was willing to work like hell to get it. I didn't read the literature at this time. Later, of course, I had to. I got mine from the AA meetings.

"Probably the most important thing I learned initially was that I couldn't control anything but myself. If change was to occur, it would have to be me that changed. I was told that the same person would drink. I didn't want to drink, so I welcomed the program into my life. To this day, I don't know what goes on at the meetings that attracts me and makes me feel so good. In retrospect, I know that I have learned a good deal, but I don't know how or which meetings are responsible for what part of what I have learned. It's been years, but I still hit six or seven meetings a week."

Although the subject and type of meetings vary, a certain amount of information is constant. Slogans become the punch lines of jokes as well as finding application in the lives of the thousands who attend AA meetings throughout the country. The philosophy is simple and unabashedly corny being laced with bromides such as "One day at a time," "There but for the grace of God," "Easy does it," and so on. What emerges from the mix of bromides, subjects, and sharing is an ordering of priorities and a sense that things are going to be pretty much the way they should be for the individual. It isn't so much that what is heard is new, but at a meeting, it all seems so applicable. Perhaps more important, the membership, particularly the newcomers, are receptive to change in the most fundamental aspects of their lives. They have to be. Their lives depend on these changes.

The vehicle that delivers the majority of the program to the membership is meetings. Suggestions about how to handle change and the sober life emerge from the collective experience of the group. The basis of this experience is the Twelve Steps and the Twelve Traditions of the program of AA. The process of working the program is simple, so simple that it is frequently obscured by overinterpretation. The leavening in this mix is discipline. Note, however, that this discipline is not directed at "not drinking," for that is a by-product of having the discipline to work the program. Discipline is, therefore, the practice of carrying out the attendance, inventory, and sharing aspects of the program on a day-to-day basis with faith in its outcome.

Faith in the program is the cornerstone of a successful experience in AA. This is most effectively demonstrated by what the fellowship refers to as "the power of example." In the Traditions, AA is defined as a program of attraction rather than of promotion. Living examples of sobriety are present in every meeting. Anniversaries of sobriety are celebrated with cakes and descriptions of life in the program. Those unfortunate persons who, for one reason or another, try to drink again also serve as examples. Many return to report that attempts at controlled drinking do not work; things just get worse. The alcoholic cannot drink. At the meetings one hears over and over "One day at a time" and "It is the first drink that gets you drunk."

The first meeting is often a surprise. "Alcoholics don't look like that," one member recalling his first meeting remarked. "I could not believe that these people were drunks. They were clean and well dressed, standing around drinking coffee, talking, and laughing. I was sweating and angry, ready to condemn and certain that I didn't belong—but didn't belong anywhere else either. I kept waiting for something dramatic to happen. It didn't. The meeting began in an orderly manner and a perfect stranger told my story. I thought

I had been set up. I thought that the whole thing had been staged as a way of getting me to stop drinking. After a while of people sharing their feelings and experiences, a curious thing happened. I began to feel I was where I belonged. I didn't know these people, but I was more like them and they were more like me than any group I had ever been around. They seemed genuinely glad to see me. I felt overwhelmed by emotion—indefinable emotion.

"When I went home later, I couldn't say why, but I felt better. I guess what I felt was hope. I didn't know what was in my future, but I knew where I was going tomorrow night. I was going to a meeting. I felt I could stay away from a drink for twenty-four hours—until then. If I got worried or wanted to talk something out to avoid a drink in that period of time, I had several phone numbers given to me at the meetings. Help would be there if I needed it. I've been sober for a while. Now, I take newcomers to meetings. I go to seven or eight a week. I needed them to get sober; now I need them to stay sober. I want to be there when a newcomer needs a phone number."

Fellowship

It seems like a paradox. People obsessed with alcohol, who build their lives around booze, lose that obsession by gathering daily with people equally obsessed. There is a lot of laughing at AA meetings. What people laugh at, however, is frequently arcane. At one meeting, a twenty-four-year-old college student chaired, describing his short but active period of drinking and taking drugs. The room filled with loud, explosive laughter as he described falls, broken bones, two school dismissals, and four automobile accidents in one night. He talked about anguish, fear, hopelessness, and isolation. His story was lived in part by all and ended well. It ended in hope at an AA meeting. AA meetings are the place for this kind of sharing. The young man in question was not trying to impress anybody with the severity of his problem; his active membership in AA demonstrated that to all.

Unlike in other social circumstances, where age is viewed as a guarantor of wisdom, it is assumed that everyone in an AA meeting has something to learn from the individual chairing, regardless of who or what that individual is. In some ways, this college student's age was measured by his years of sobriety, and people many times his senior were noted paying close attention to his description of his program for living sober. He appeared to know more about that than many of the chronologically older newcomers in the room. He had one advantage over a lot of young people who find themselves obsessed with alcohol or caught up in the combination of taking drugs and drinking. His mother was an alcoholic and had been in AA for fifteen or more years. She did not insist that her son go to meetings when she knew he was in trouble. She did not preach to him; she did not talk about his unwillingness to see the example of his mother's sobriety. To the contrary, she waited and watched for that curious combination of remorse, self-hatred, fear, and insight called the "bottom" to occur. When it did, she invited him to a meeting. He was fortunate. He has not had a drink since. It should be noted that intergenerational family membership is not unusual in AA. A lot of people describe AA meetings for them as a kind of gathering of the clan where they see fathers, mothers, sisters, brothers, cousins, aunts, uncles, and more distant relatives.

Sharing

Sharing at a meeting can illuminate the most intimate or humiliating details of one's life. Things that would never be shared in anything other than the most private of circumstances are aired for a large number of comparative strangers. A membership knows all about each other; they share love and compassion but seldom last names. Open meetings still are not the place for confessions; intimate details perhaps, but not confessions. The latter is the thrust of the Fourth and the Fifth Steps. An important part of meetings, nonetheless, is the sharing of intense or emotionally charged deeds or feelings. Meetings are permissive of sharing, eliciting compassion in response. It is not unusual in meetings to have people openly weep at their initial confession of alcoholism. It is not a sad event, nor does it draw a good deal of attention. The significance of admission and the emotional impact of that admission lie in its implied surrender for the individual. In AA sobriety and change begin with surrender. We see this in the First Step: "We admitted we were powerless over alcohol—that our lives have become unmanageable."

Another subject guaranteed to strike a respondent chord is methods of drinking and/or symptoms. Tales of sheer volume will not impress this group. Early morning drinking will not surprise this group. Binges of monumental proportions will draw raised eyebrows at best. This group has done it all. They do, however, pay attention to arcane methods of drinking or unusual rituals associated with certain kinds of drinking patterns. One gentleman reported, for example, that when he drank in the morning he was careful to mix his vodka with either fresh grapefruit juice or freshly squeezed orange juice. A self-confessed health enthusiast, he reasoned that because alcohol washed vitamins out of the body, he would mix his alcohol with the freshest of ingredients and take large amounts of vitamin supplements. In this way he could drink without becoming vitamin poor. A jogger, he carried two things with him while running between five and fifteen miles a day: a small flask of vodka and Gatorade. He washed his vitamin pills down with beer, which brought about vomiting and diarrhea. He had physical aches and pains typical of the middle or later stages of alcoholism. He switched to what he called organic alcohol as a natural cure. You guessed it; he drank wine by the gallon.

As this story unfolded, the people in the meeting nodded their heads and laughed at the reasoning that could allow a college graduate with a professional degree to justify continued drinking. As the man said himself, "I would not stop drinking." He also said that when he first came into the program, he had difficulties with the Steps that talked about returning him to sanity. He maintained that he was not insane. He did not have any emotional or psychological problems; he just drank too much.

After a few months of sobriety, as the fog gradually began to lift from his mind, he could look at logic such as he described in the meetings and realize that this is a good definition of insanity. He defined *insanity* as the maintenance of behavior guaranteed to cause self-destruction—or the continuance of behavior such as drinking in the face of certain knowledge that continued drinking will kill you. In a particularly subdued manner, he said that throughout his drinking life he felt he was drinking voluntarily. He took a drink when he wanted to; he felt that he drank in the morning because he wanted to or because he was sick. He honestly believed that he continued drinking because he wanted to drink, even after watching himself pass blood in his urine in the morning. When he got sober, he was able to take an honest look at the obsessive nature of his drinking and see that he was not drinking voluntarily. He was compelled to drink. It was necessary for something outside of him to intervene to interrupt that compulsion.

A university professor reported his drinking in a straightforward, deadpan delivery. He said he was by nature a compulsive person given to great order and organization. He kept lists of things and never threw out anything. His work in research reflected this kind of obsession. When he began to worry about his daily intake of alcohol, he began keeping accurate records of it. (When people begin to wonder whether or not they have a drinking problem, they usually do.) His concerns grew out of a litany of physical symptoms that were typical of alcoholism. He began maintenance drinking systematically and kept a journal of his intake, supplemented by pills. His description of his drinking career began with a ten-minute reading from journal notations such as "8:30—2 ounces of vodka, 86 proof, relief felt, shaking continues unabated, 2 Valium," and so on. Times and amounts were listed daily.

The group's reaction to this was absolute hilarity. Some remarked that they could not write when they were drinking; others said that they could not write until after they stopped drinking. It was not the amount of alcohol consumed but the method of counting that was of interest to the meeting. Like most AA stories, however, this one ended on a positive note. Here was the professor chairing an AA meeting, sober for quite some time, sharing his strength and hope with the group and making clear another aspect of alcoholism. The people at that meeting were not all list keepers, but alcohol had made them all crazy in one way or another. When they sobered up, they stopped being crazy.

In many ways, the purpose of an AA meeting is to remind alcoholics where they came from. It is easy to forget the pain and incredible list of symptoms that finally drive a person to join Alcoholics Anonymous. For this reason, people chairing meetings often describe the physical symptoms that finally convinced them that their alcoholism was acute and demanded treatment or intervention. After listening to a number of drunk-a-logues, one draws the impression that it is not the severity of symptoms that finally frightens the alcoholic person into seeking help. To the contrary, the alcoholic's response to a symptom is to adjust to whatever physical or psychological inconvenience the alcohol imposes. There is a willingness to do anything but stop drinking.

The physical symptoms are simply part of the entire physical, psychological and spiritual package that drives alcoholics to submission and finally forces them to seek help. Morning tales of vomiting, shaking, sweating, diarrhea, passing blood in the urine, memory lapses, falling down—even such things as loss of the use of limbs through alcohol's attack on the nervous system—do not frighten so much as provide a way for group members to identify with each other. Some have experienced all of these symptoms. Some have experienced only a few. One thing is clear, however; the symptoms do not exist as individual, unique experiences. To the contrary, they are the inevitable result of drinking alcohol. So, for some, a discussion of symptoms is a walk down memory lane and a good reminder of where they came from. For others, it is a harbinger of the future and a clear statement of the inevitability of things to come if they continue to drink or return to drinking.

The point of all of this sharing is identification; it tells the alcoholic that he or she is not unique. Although many and varied, alcoholics share a number of things in common. They are not as bad as they think they are. Although each begins involvement in AA by reaching a bottom, bottoms differ. Although they have all ridden the elevator of alcoholism, each has gotten off on a different floor. The meetings provide a way of looking at the entire existential experience of alcoholism, thereby broadening the individual's perspective on what he or she has experienced. The meetings, therefore, tend to lessen feelings of "Why me?"

To end his sharing, Frank concludes: "If we can identify with things others have done, we benefit. If we share things that we have done, we benefit. As alcoholics in AA, we share a common bond. If we hear things we have not done, we know what we can look forward to. It is like a paint-by-the-numbers picture of alcoholism. Each of us paints in a part of the picture, and all of us get a total view of the impact of the disease on our lives. It is as the book says: 'we will see how our experience can benefit others.'[19] As alcoholics in AA, we do not tell our stories to satisfy the curious or with a sense of bravado. We try to share our past so that we can put it in order, in perspective, and get about the business of living our lives sober."

2

A MATTER OF DEFINITION

Basic Definitions

Alcohol abuse is a significant social problem. Its dimensions are almost beyond measure. Public policy and treatment strategies depend on how alcohol abuse is defined, which is more complex than one would imagine.

Enoch Gordis, examining the scope of the alcohol- and drug-related problems in the United States, estimated that nearly 14 million adults meet the diagnostic criteria for alcohol addiction or abuse.[1] One of every four children under the age of eighteen in this country will have some kind of contact with alcoholism in the family. "Some twenty to forty percent of patients in urban hospital beds are being treated for health problems associated with alcohol use. This means that in any given city hospital, almost one half of the patient population may be there because of alcohol use. Other consequences of alcohol abuse include deterioration of the family unit and costs associated with police, courts, jails and unemployment. Altogether the consequences of alcohol abuse and dependence are estimated to be $185 billion and 100,000 deaths annually."[2] Culturally, alcohol is integral, prescribed for sadness and celebration alike. Can we identify those who are vulnerable to addiction to psychoactive substances? Can we identify those already addicted to psychoactive substances? How can we best deal with the problems connected with such addictions?

How we define a thing determines how we think about and deal with it. The designation of the etiology of alcoholism suggests not only the parameters of its study but also, by implication, the appropriate way to address the problem or treat the alcoholic.

Cultural Differences

To understand cultural differences in definitions of normal and abusive drinking, we must consider relevant social, political, and legal perspectives. Even these perspectives do not result in categories that are mutually inclusive and exclusive. In the United States, for example, mores governing all aspects of alcohol intake vary greatly from region to region. In each geographic area, additional variations occur between social classes.

Alcohol-related legal issues also vary in definition, region to region. Generally, alcohol abuse, such as evidenced in public drunkenness or drunken driving, is condemned. Yet public intoxication is expected at outdoor music venues or citywide events like Mardi Gras and football or baseball games. College settings are frequently tolerant of drinking and drunken behavior, but even these settings have their limits. Legal access to alcohol is limited by age in the United States, but enforcement varies from region to region.

The social definition of alcohol abuse and alcoholism is perhaps easier to understand. It simply defines alcohol abuse in terms of its impact on an individual and on related systems such as work performance and loss of work. It also takes into account the medical costs of treating alcoholism, and the social costs of alcohol-related violence and family deterioration. It is clear that different social contexts result in very different definitions of what constitutes alcoholism.[3] Of necessity, treatment modalities require specific definition. I examine three of these definitions, concluding with the AA perspective. It is instructive to consider the similarities and differences of all of these models.

The *Diagnostic and Statistical Manual of Mental Diseases* (*DSM IV-TR*) basic criteria for alcohol dependence and alcohol abuse are the same as those for substance dependence and substance abuse. The basic criteria for substance dependence are:

A maladaptive pattern of substance use, leading to clinically significant impairment or distress, as manifested by three (or more) of the following, occurring at any time in the same 12-month period:

(1) tolerance, as defined by either of the following:

(a) a need for markedly increased amounts of the substance to achieve intoxication or desired effect

(b) markedly diminished effect with continued use of the same amount of the substance

(2) withdrawal, as manifested by either of the following:

(a) the characteristic withdrawal syndrome for the substance . . .

(b) the same (or a closely related) substance is taken to relieve or avoid withdrawal symptoms

(3) the substance is often taken in larger amounts or over a longer period than was intended

(4) there is a persistent desire or unsuccessful efforts to cut down or control substance use

(5) a great deal of time is spent in activities necessary to obtain the substance (e.g., visiting multiple doctors or driving long distances), use the substance (e.g., chain smoking), or recover from its effects

(6) important social, occupational, or recreational activities are given up or reduced because of substance use

(7) the substance use is continued despite knowledge of having a persistent physical or psychological problem that is likely to have been caused or exacerbated by the substance (e.g., current cocaine use despite recognition of cocaine-induced depression, or continued drinking despite recognition that an ulcer was made worse by alcohol consumption)[4]

The basic criteria for substance abuse are:

A. A maladaptive pattern of substance use leading to clinically significant impairment or distress, as manifested by one (or more) of the following, occurring within a 12-month period:

(1) recurrent substance use resulting in a failure to fulfill major role obligations at work, school, or home (e.g., repeated absences or poor work performance related to substance use; substance-related absences, suspensions, or expulsions from school; neglect of children or household)

(2) recurrent substance use in situations in which it is physically hazardous (e.g., driving an automobile or operating a machine when impaired by substance use)

(3) recurrent substance-related legal problems (e.g., arrests for substance-related disorderly conduct)

(4) continued substance use despite having persistent or recurrent social or interpersonal problems caused or exacerbated by the effects of the

substance (e.g., arguments with spouse about the consequences of intoxication, physical fights)

B. The symptoms have never met the criteria for Substance Dependence for this class of substance.[5]

The *International Classification of Diseases,* 10th revision (*ICD-10*), states, "Identification of the psychoactive substance should be based on as many sources of information as possible. These include self-report data, analysis of blood and other body fluids, characteristic physical and psychological symptoms, clinical signs and behaviour and other evidence such as a drug being in the patient's possession or reports from informed third parties."[6] *Acute intoxication* is defined as "a condition that follows the administration of a psychoactive substance resulting in disturbances in level of consciousness, cognition, perception, affect or behaviour, or other psycho-physiological functions and responses. The disturbances are directly related to the acute pharmacological effects of the substance and resolve with time, with complete recovery, except where tissue damage or other complications have arisen." *Harmful use* is defined as "a pattern of psychoactive substance use that is causing damage to health. The damage may be physical (as in cases of hepatitis, from the self-administration of injected psychoactive substances) or mental (e.g., episodes of depressive disorder secondary to heavy consumption of alcohol)." It defines *dependence syndrome* as "a cluster of behavioural, cognitive, and physiological phenomena that develop after repeated substance use and that typically include a strong desire to take the drug, difficulties in controlling its use, persisting in its use despite harmful consequences, a higher priority given to drug use than to other activities and obligations, increased tolerance, and sometimes a physical withdrawal state." The manual continues describing the withdrawal state and delirium in much the same way the *DSM IV-TR* does. It also includes a description of *psychotic disorder:* "A cluster of psychotic phenomena that occur during or following psychoactive substance use but that are not explained on the basis of acute intoxication alone and do not form a part of the withdrawal state."[7] In the case of the alcoholic person, hallucinosis, paranoia, and jealousy are specifically noted. It also notes the amnesic syndrome typically defined as "blackouts" among alcoholics in AA. In many ways, these definitions are commonly understood.

E. Mansell Pattison and Edward Kaufman suggest that misuse of alcohol is often defined by its adverse consequences. They note that the definition of alcohol abuse is dependent on the mores that pertain to given systems. For example, alcohol abuse at a party might be defined as simply being overly exuberant. They note that alcohol is frequently used as an excuse for bad behavior. They point out, however, that "in abuse patterns there is a chronic, recurrent use of alcohol with both acute and chronic adverse consequences. Physiological and/or psychological dependence on alcohol is established. Such abuse can be socially acceptable as in heavy social drinking: the use may be acceptable as in drinking alcohol per se, but the consequent behavior may be unacceptable; or both use and consequence may be socially unacceptable."[8] Particularly interesting is their description of psychic dependence resulting from alcohol being psychoactive: "It changes the conscious state of the consumer in one way or another. It does not matter much what change in consciousness is produced. The alcohol dependent person relies on a change in consciousness to cope more effectively with self and to experience reality. Thus alcohol dependent people commonly also switch to other types of drugs and develop mixed drug and alcohol dependence. The alcohol dependent person has a psychological reliance on the psychic effect of the drug to produce an altered state of consciousness."[9]

No one sets out to develop a dependence on drugs or alcohol. The authors suggest that perhaps some people vary in vulnerability as they experience social milieus that are accepting of drug or alcohol use for either celebration or problem solving. They also logically point out that "persons who might otherwise be highly vulnerable to developing alcohol dependence may avoid such a possibility through total avoidance of alcohol use."[10] Others have suggested the division of alcohol users into types. An individual of type 1 characteristically uses alcohol intermittently by choice for the purpose of obtaining or enhancing pleasure. A type 2 individual uses alcohol to relieve distress, mitigate a painful emotional state, or alleviate anxiety. A type 3 individual uses alcohol to manage the difficulties and distresses of everyday life. For this person, alcohol is the lubricant for the very gears of life. This could be a typology of alcohol use as well as a typology of alcohol users.[11]

Other categories of alcoholics are defined by use. One that comes to mind is the *maintenance* drinker, defined as a person who drinks continuously to maintain a level of alcohol in the body that allows the person, by self-description, to feel "normal." Maintenance drinkers are frequently quite functional, successfully negotiating daily life without undue attention being paid to their drinking. Another recognized category is the *binge* drinker, who abstains from alcohol for relatively long periods of time between drinks. When drinking begins, it is characteristically an all-consuming activity resulting in a continuous state of drunkenness. The binge ends when one of two events takes place: the individual runs out of liquor or money and is not physically able to obtain any more alcohol, or the individual becomes so toxic that he or she is finally taken to the hospital for treatment. Characteristically, once a binge begins, the individual is unable to interrupt the drinking process. An *episodic* drinker is sometimes distinguished from the binge drinker on the basis of the length of time between episodes of heavy drinking. An episodic drinker may go many months or even years between binges.

Yet another category is the *social* drinker (a term supposedly invented by alcoholics). The social drinker has no problems with alcohol. He or she can drink or not drink. The person experiences no compulsion to continue drinking after having had a drink. At AA meetings, one frequently hears complaints about wives or husbands who at parties are able to have a drink, put it down, forget where it is, and not go back to it. For the alcoholic person, this behavior is confusing. It should be noted that anyone might experience any or all of these patterns of drinking in his or her drinking career. The heterogeneous nature of the phenomenon makes it difficult to develop categories of alcohol abuse or dependence that are mutually inclusive or exclusive.

It is impossible to consider definitions of the alcoholic person without considering the work of E. M. Jellinek. He was the first director of the Yale Summer School of Alcohol Studies and the first editor of the *Quarterly Journal of Studies on Alcohol.* He wrote *The Disease Concept of Alcoholism.*[12] It was Jellinek's position that the core of alcoholism was an inability to control drinking once the process had begun.[13] Jellinek's most famous contribution to the field was his delineation of the evolution of alcoholism in the individual, sometimes referred to as Jellinek's Curve. The stages are listed below.

JELLINEK CHART OF ALCOHOL ADDICTION

Prealcoholic Phase
    a. Occasional relief drinking
    b. Constant relief drinking
    c. Increase in alcohol tolerance

Prodromal Phase

    1. Onset of blackouts

    2. Surreptitious drinking

    3. Anticipatory drinking

    4. Gulping drinks

    5. Guilt feelings

    6. Avoiding reference to alcohol

    7. Frequent blackouts

Crucial Phase

    8. Loss of control

    9. Rationalized drinking

    10. Social pressures

    11. Grandiose behavior

    12. Aggressive behavior

    13. Persistent remorse

    14. Periods of total abstinence

    15. Changing drinking pattern

    16. Dropping friends

    17. Quitting jobs

    18. Behavior becomes alcohol-centered

    19. Loss of outside interests

    20. Reinterpretation of interpersonal relations

    21. Marked self-pity

    22. Geographic escape

    23. Change in family habits

    24. Unreasonable resentments

    25. Protecting supply

    26. Nutritional neglect

    27. First hospitalization (alcoholism)

    28. Decreased sexual drive

    29. Alcoholic jealousy

    30. Regular morning drinking

Chronic Phase

    31. Onset of benders

    32. Marked ethical deterioration

    33. Impairment of thinking

34. Alcoholic psychoses
35. Drinking down (socially)
36. Drinking technical products
37. Loss of alcohol tolerance
38. Indefinable fears
39. Tremors
40. Psychomotor inhibition
41. Obsessive drinking
42. Religious needs
43. Admitting defeat[14]

These definitions do not appear to be essentially different, for they all focus on the outcome of alcohol abuse. In his focus on social career, however, Jellinek's work comes closest to a longitudinal understanding of the phenomena. Anyone can be located on his scale of events and severity, regardless of age of onset or the rate at which the abuse accelerates. It is both descriptive and predictive.

Multivariate Syndrome

Some definitions of alcoholism primarily focus on psychological aspects. Others focus on the sociocultural context in which the behavior manifests itself, while still others focus on biological factors interacting with both the social and psychological aspects of the individual. Other definitions identify more than one cause of alcoholism. They focus on alcoholism in its diversity, referring to it as a multivariate syndrome. "That is, there are multiple patterns of dysfunctional alcohol use that occur in multiple types of personalities, with multiple combinations of adverse consequences, with multiple prognoses, that may require different types of treatment interventions."[15] This particular definition of alcoholism seems to focus on the context of habituation. In this definition, there are many roads leading to alcoholism. Each circumstance or "road" contains influences that structure the individual's choices regarding alcohol intake.

The multivariate approach to diagnosis "leads one to consider alcoholism as a syndrome. . . . Medical dictionaries define *syndrome* as a group or set of concurrent symptoms that together can be considered a disease. Note that considering alcoholism as a syndrome does not vitiate alcoholism as a disease, for medical practice in general deals with many syndromes that are not specific diseases."[16] The following are the assumptions of the multivariate alcoholism syndrome.

1. There is a unitary phenomenon that can be identified as alcoholism despite variations; there is a distinct entity.
2. Alcoholics or pre-alcoholics are essentially different from nonalcoholics.
3. Alcoholics experience an irresistible physical craving for alcohol or an overwhelming psychological compulsion to drink.
4. Alcoholics develop a process of loss of control over initiation of drinking and/or inability to stop drinking.
5. Alcoholism is a permanent and irreversible condition.
6. Alcoholism is a progressive disease that follows an inexorable development through a series of more or less destructive phases.[17]

This model duplicates the formal and informal definitions used in the literature of alcoholism and the meetings of Alcoholics Anonymous. Common usage in AA, however, defines alcoholism as a disease rather than a multivariate syndrome. Yet I think the AA response to this difference would be, "So what?" The thrust of AA is not to discuss the etiology of alcoholism but rather to treat it. Note that the AA definition of alcoholism is binary. One is either alcoholic or not; there is no middle ground. I discuss the AA definition of alcoholism and its implications and complications in the program later in this chapter.

Disease?

While AA members generally do not particularly care about the scientific accuracy of their definition of alcoholism as a disease, others do. In fact, a controversy is reflected in the literature considering the various definitions of alcoholism. The idea of alcohol as a disease relies on an assumption, according to Paul R. McHugh and Phillip R. Slavney, that "diseases are afflictions in which an abnormality of a bodily part provokes the affliction's characteristic symptoms, signs, and course. This disease-provoking bodily abnormality may be one of structure (such as tumors and infarcts) or one of function (such as excesses or deficiencies in neuronal activity or endocrine secretion). The symptoms and signs of the patients with a disease often indicate the nature of the bodily abnormality, but the analysis of blood chemistries, radiological images, electrocardiograms, and so forth, is usually necessary to specify it. . . . Disease reasoning, in fact, combines a categorical method for differentiating human afflictions, ultimately distinguishing them by their underlying abnormalities."[18] McHugh and Slavney indicate that the disease reasoning leads to a path that tracks down causes. They feel, therefore, that the disease concept links etiology with a categorization of the phenomena that is both inclusive and exclusive. Given this definition, our present state of medical knowledge would not allow us to categorize alcoholism as a disease. As McHugh and Slavney state, "Like all explanatory methods, disease reasoning has clear advantages and disadvantages."[19] Perhaps multivariate syndrome is a better choice.

Edgar Nace, in *The Treatment of Alcoholism,* discusses Pattison and Kaufman's perspective on the multivariate syndrome:

> This concept recognizes the diversity inherent in the phenomena of alcoholism, including multiple patterns of use and abuse of alcohol, multiple interacting etiological variables, and variations in the populations of individuals with alcohol problems. The advantage of viewing alcoholism as a syndrome is the recognition that there are many pathways to alcoholism. This conceptualization contrasts with efforts to delineate alcoholism as a strictly biological process, genetically determined and unfolding over the course of a lifetime with a characteristic sequence and a predictable outcome. It also contrasts with efforts that attempt to explain alcoholism as the outgrowth of a specific personality type. No inherent contradictions need exist between considering alcoholism as a disease or syndrome.[20]

Nace goes on, "Disease is an applicable term because of the commonality of psychological dependence and related phenomena . . . which exist across the multivariate pattern progressions and etiologies. In other words, regardless of how one acquires alcohol dependence or which symptoms predominate at the subjective level, the disorder manifests a characteristic influence on thinking and behavior." Nace concurs that there are no proven distinctions in brain or other organ functioning between the alcoholic and the nonalcoholic. He notes that the patterns of brain and organ damage commonly associated with alcoholism are secondary to that disease. He further suggests that our inability to locate a defining state of biology that would separate the alcoholic from the nonalcoholic is a function of the state of our science rather than of the proposition that the etiology of alcoholism is not biological. He is also aware of the social and political aspects of the definition of alcoholism. "The ambivalence and confusion over the acceptance of alcoholism as a disease may lie partly in an uncertainty as to what the disease of alcoholism actually is. If we had a metabolic explanation for the etiology of alcoholism, a greater acceptance of the disease concept and improved service might occur, but we have no such explanation, and most physicians give a vague 'lip service' without a sense of conviction to the disease concept. The fragility of our acceptance of the disease concept renders us vulnerable to the idea that the alcoholic is engaging in unacceptable behavior willingly."[21] This is also a paradox long familiar to members of Alcoholics Anonymous. In AA it is frequently stated that alcoholics are not bad people but are sick people trying to get well. It is a contention in AA that people are responsible for the content of their behavior. The thrust of analysis of that behavior attempts to get to what caused the behavior other than choice. The behavior is seen as motivated by or driven by the effect of alcohol on the individual. As AA members note, "Drinking alcohol makes us crazy. Is it any wonder that our behavior is crazy?" The common denominator is alcoholism. Nace makes sense of the controversy in the following manner: "Understanding the disease of alcoholism will not come from the observation of external manifestations of alcohol use. Nor does the physician need to wait for a biochemical explanation in order to accept the concept of disease. Acceptance can emerge as one comprehends the subjective experience of the alcoholic patient and the impact of alcohol on the thinking, motivation and personality functioning of the alcohol dependent individual. Six constructs make up the essential phenomenon of alcoholism: psychological dependence on a chemical, craving, loss of control, personality regression, denial and conflicted behavior."[22]

Whether or not you agree with the disease model or the multivariate syndrome model, both recognize the patterns of hereditary transmission of vulnerability to alcoholism.

Genetics

On October 15, 1999, Enoch Gordis, M.D., director of the National Institute on Alcohol Abuse and Alcoholism, presented a paper, "Improving the Old, Embracing the New: Implications of Alcohol Research for Future Practice," at the Eighth Doris Siegel Memorial Colloquium at the Mount Sinai Hospital in New York City.[23] Gordis emphasized that alcohol research has two important goals: to evaluate existing therapies for treating alcoholism and to increase understanding of the biology of alcoholism. The latter, he felt, was important because it helped pinpoint medications to prevent alcohol abuse problems or to improve treatment outcomes.

New neuroscience techniques have led to an increased understanding of how alcohol's actions in the brain are related to the phenomenon of addiction and new imaging techniques have permitted scientists to study alcohol's effects on the brain and to link these effects to behaviors in ways not even possible just a few years ago. Finally genetics researchers are using both animal and human genetics techniques to identify the genes that confer vulnerability to alcoholism and developing ways to apply this information to clinical populations. As a result of increased understanding of the biology of alcohol dependence future clinicians will need to understand not just the traditional behavioral nuances of alcoholism treatment but the biology of alcohol dependence as well.[24]

In his definition of alcoholism, Gordis parallels those found in the *DSM IV-TR* and the *ICD-10*. He suggests that 8 to 10 percent of adults show the various symptoms of alcoholism (alcohol dependence). He notes that this 10 percent demonstrate physical dependence on alcohol, are sick when they stop drinking (withdrawal), need more and more alcohol to produce the same effect (that is, they develop a tolerance to alcohol), and, once they begin drinking, have no way of controlling how much they drink. They also manifest a craving that is thought to be a major factor in relapse. Gordis notes that these mechanisms appear to be involved in vulnerability to dependency, and he suggests that this is why only a minority of people who begin to drink alcohol get into trouble with it. Of course, he also says that effective research in this area is needed. Defining the relationship of alcoholism to genetic research, he remarks that perhaps 50 to 60 percent of the vulnerability to developing alcoholism is genetic. This finding is based on human population studies conducted during the 1970s which focused on twins and adoptees. No specific genes have been identified in conferring this vulnerability.

In twin studies, identical twins are compared with fraternal twins. In identical twins all of the genes are the same; fraternal twins only share one half of their genes. To find out about their vulnerability to alcoholism scientists ask the following questions: Given that the first member of the twin pair is alcoholic, what are the odds that the other member is alcoholic? The answer is two out of three—about 65 percent—that an identical twin will be alcoholic if his twin pair is alcoholic. In the case of fraternal twins who share only half of their genes the odds of the second twin being alcoholic was only about 3 out of 10. This tells us two things. First, it tells us there is a genetic role in the vulnerability to alcoholism. Second, it tells us that genes are not the whole story. If they were the whole story, the odds of twins being alcoholic would be 100 percent. These findings set the stage for the considerable progress that we have made in understanding the genetics of alcoholism.[25]

Beginning in 1989, the National Institute on Alcohol Abuse and Alcoholism (NIAAA) supported a collaborative, multisite study that assessed individuals from multigenerational families with a prevalence of alcoholism.

Each of these families contained at least three first degree relatives with alcohol dependence. Using a variety of cutting-edge tools and techniques from molecular biology, neurochemistry, statistics and clinical research, COGA (Collaborative Study on the Genetics of Alcoholism) scientists found highly suggestive evidence for chromosomal "hot spots" (areas of potential linkage to alcohol dependence) on chromosomes 1 and 2 and more modest evidence on chromosomes 4 and 7. In addition, locations for the genes involved in the expression of evoked potential responses, a high risk mark for alcoholism, were also identified. These findings bring us a step closer to finding the genes underlying the genetic vulnerability to this chronic disease.[26]

A number of other factors also influence the possibility of someone developing a drinking problem or alcoholism. A study undertaken by the NIAAA, called the National Longitudinal Alcohol Epidemiological Survey (NLAES), found that the earlier a young person begins to drink, the greater the odds are that he or she will become alcoholic as an adult. "This is the case without respect to a family history of alcoholism or gender, or a variety of other indicators that we normally look at to determine what influences the risk of disease. Looking at this sample of 42,000 people, we discovered that the risks of becoming an alcoholic, if you start drinking before the age of 15, are forty percent. If drinking does not begin until age 18 or 20, this risk is reduced to about 10%, which is about the national prevalence of alcohol use problems."[27] To assess genetic risk, one needs to examine the gene/environment interaction. Genes are not destiny.

Philip R. Reilly, examining the relationship of genes to alcoholism, suggests that alcoholism is a complex disease difficult to define and hard to study. "In developing diagnostic criteria to define alcoholism, experts have been forced to rely on measurements of the impact of consumption on the individual's ability to maintain his or her normal activities. For five decades, the core concept of alcoholism as a disease has been that an alcoholic is a person who is physiologically dependent on alcohol and cannot function without having nearly constant access to it."[28] Reilly estimates the probability of becoming an alcoholic in the United States as 5 to 7 percent in men, but only 0.5 to 1 percent in women. He notes also that alcoholism runs in families and that a voluminous literature reports that children have a higher risk of becoming alcoholic if one or more parent is alcoholic. They are also statistically more likely to have siblings that are alcoholic. Reilly cites twin studies, including a "1998 study of a Finnish group of severe alcoholics (166 alcoholics with criminal records arising out of antisocial behavior while they were inebriated, 261 unaffected relatives and 213 controls) [which] found evidence linking a variant in the serotonin receptor gene (HTRIB) to risk for disease . . . When compared to the general population, the children of alcoholics and the siblings of alcoholics have a three to five fold greater risk for the disease. For those with a strong family history of alcohol problems the best approach is the simplest. Abstinence is a perfect prevention of alcoholism."[29]

The AA Perspective on Definition

A major influence on the AA founders, Dr. William Silkworth joined the staff at Towns Hospital in New York with the intention of treating alcoholics. By the time he met Bill Wilson, Dr. Silkworth had already formulated his theory of allergy. Later, in a 1937 article "Alcoholism as a Manifestation of an Allergy" in the *Medical Record,* he likened the alcoholic's allergic state to the plight of the hay fever patient who gradually becomes sensitized to certain types of pollen.

Dr. Silkworth described his theory as follows: "We believe . . . that the action of alcohol on . . . chronic alcoholics [is] a manifestation of an allergy; that the phenomenon of craving is limited to this class and never occurs in the average, temperate drinker. These allergic types can never safely use alcohol in any form at all; and once having formed the habit and found they cannot break it, once having lost their self confidence, their reliance upon things human, their problems pile up on them and become astonishingly difficult to solve."[30] Bill Wilson was intrigued by this unique theory and came to believe that alcoholism was a combination of a physical allergy and the compulsion to drink. Silkworth's definition of alcoholism as biological rather than a moral lapse or a function of choice laid the groundwork for AA's philosophy of defining alcoholism as a disease or physically rooted phenomenon.[31] Certainly, early members of AA were well aware of the family transmission theory of alcoholism, and the biological model made their observations all the more understandable and related to the unique framework within which Alcoholics Anonymous addressed treatment.

For whatever reason, alcoholism defined as a disease is common currency in AA. This definition pertains regardless of the contradictions or paradoxes associated with it. Members describe themselves as having alcoholism. The treatment is abstinence supported by the program. The "disease" cannot be cured, but it can be arrested. I think it is fair to say that people in AA, at all levels, ultimately have no interest in the etiology of alcoholism. Their definition of alcoholism as a disease is also intentionally political. Defining alcoholism as a disease takes it out of the realm of moral choice and casts it as a compulsion/obsession rooted in biology. The vocabulary of this explanation includes assumptions that the hereditary transmission of alcoholism is proof of its biological roots and that alcoholics somehow synthesize alcohol differently from nonalcoholics. For those in AA, the difference between the alcoholic and the nonalcoholic lies in the reaction to alcohol. The alcoholic's obsession and the compulsive nature of his or her drinking defines the person in most contexts. For this reason, nonalcoholics have such a difficult time understanding the alcoholic. They simply don't have the same relationship to alcohol.

A member of AA for thirty years or so described this phenomenon in a conversation. "I have always had a very special relationship with alcohol. I didn't know this because, both in my family and in the range of my social experience, people didn't talk about or ask questions about anyone's relationship to alcohol. It was assumed that you didn't have a relationship with alcohol. It was assumed in my social setting that everyone had the same relationship with alcohol. From the time I first drank at eleven years of age, I thought about alcohol and when I would drink again. Early social activities were structured around the availability of alcohol at those events. I don't mean I got drunk every time I went out or for that matter that I drank in any way that could be distinguished from those of my friends. It was simply that I thought about and weighed the importance of alcohol in the events that I went to. If growing up in America has rights of passage connected with alcohol, and I think it does, all of my rights of passage occurred very early. Throughout my early years, I assumed that everybody felt the same way that I did about alcohol. I thought that they too focused on its abilities to act as a social lubricant and as a way of temporizing with the pressures and anxieties of the drive to succeed in this culture. It wasn't until I was in trouble with alcohol and had been for some time that I came to AA and found that most people do not have this kind of a relationship with alcohol. As a matter of fact, it is my opinion that this relationship is unique to the alcoholic and perhaps one of our defining characteristics. It made sense to me that my relationship to alcohol was based on a biological difference between myself and nonalcoholics. I had no other explanation for it. I think that explanation helped me understand why it was so difficult to stop drinking and why the model of total abstinence made sense to me. Since I have been in AA for a long time, I have seen people come and go. The lesson here is that AA is accurate when it says, 'One drink will get you drunk.' Whatever the difference between me and nonalcoholics, I know that one drink of alcohol will trigger whatever there is in me that compels me to drink. My only option, if I wish to maintain a viable role with my family, and society, is total abstinence."

The AA definition of alcoholism as a disease is paradoxical because everything in the AA program operates on the basis of choice. Members choose to be sober. In AA, however, choice begins after discovery. One does not choose to be an alcoholic, but one can choose how to deal with alcoholism once it is recognized.[32] Within this model, a person becomes alcoholic because his body processes alcohol differently than other people's bodies do. In the case of the alcoholic, ingestion of alcohol creates a compulsion to drink. He becomes obsessed with alcohol. The cause is in the biology. New members of AA come to believe that application of the program will arrest alcoholism in them. It becomes personal. Membership is a choice.

The Progressive Aspect of the Disease

Alcoholics Anonymous defines alcoholism as a progressive disease that persists whether or not one stops drinking, meaning that if an alcoholic person stops drinking for a period of time, then drinks again, the body's vulnerability to alcohol does not return to ground zero. The alcoholic who after a period of sobriety drinks again will never again experience the honeymoon period of early drinking. Simply put, alcoholism in the body increases in severity over time, regardless of the drinking patterns of the individual. Meetings are full of examples of this phenomenon. Is this a self-fulfilling prophecy among AA members? Does the anticipation of an outcome create that outcome? Typical of AA, the resolution to these questions is found in the experience of the membership. Betty reported at a meeting: "My mother did not drink throughout her lifetime. My father did not drink. I grew up in a home where alcohol was neither discussed nor evident. Years after I left home to establish a home of my own, I maintained close contact with my parents. My father called to ask me to come home to help him with Mother. He said she had become addicted to pills and was drinking heavily, and he worried about her health. When I returned home, I found my mother to be extremely underweight and smelling of vodka. She had become a twenty-four-hour maintenance drinker. In complaining to doctors about her inability to sleep, she had also gotten prescriptions for tranquilizers and sleeping medication, which she used to augment the impact of alcohol.

"I asked my father how Mother had gotten to this sorry state. He said he had suggested a couple of years ago that she take three or four ounces of liquor before she went to bed to help her with a long-standing sleep problem. He said in the beginning it worked very well, and then she began drinking around the clock. His description indicated that Mother had begun with a high tolerance to alcohol and within a month or two had degenerated into daily drinking and augmenting her state with tranquilizers and sleeping pills. My mother was hospitalized with what was defined as gastric problems. Whatever nutrition my mother took in, it came with vodka. I suggested that the doctor have a talk with my mother about the fact that her gastric problems were brought about by pouring vodka on an empty stomach over a period of time. The doctor was unwilling to do that and was equally unwilling to make a record of my mother's obviously alcohol-related difficulties. I spent weeks working with my mother and finally got her connected with AA. And there has been a happy outcome. Mother has been sober for the last eighteen years. She says at this point that it feels as if the events in question happened to somebody else. She attends AA meetings once in a while but has largely resumed her prior life.

"Checking into my mother's family, I discovered I had two uncles who died in the old country of alcohol-related difficulties. My mother's parents, whom I did not know, were variously involved with alcohol. My maternal grandfather apparently died of alcoholism at the age of sixty-one. Examining my father's family, I found that it too was riddled with alcoholism. Given my background and heredity, I began to understand my own alcoholism more clearly."

The point here is understood by the membership. Although the mother did not drink for the first sixty-six years of her life, when she began to drink, the impact of the alcohol was immediate and devastating. She had been alcoholic all of her life, and her disease had progressed with her age. There was no honeymoon in the drinking process, no time when drinking was controlled and pleasant. She was flagrantly alcoholic at her first ingestion of alcohol. AA meetings are peppered with this anecdotal supportive information. For the AA member, it has the ring of truth. Imbedded in the story is the idea that the condition of the individual is defined by the reaction to the alcohol. Controlled drinking for the alcoholic is impossible. The intake of alcohol guarantees the return of the compulsion to drink. Once our storyteller's mother began to drink, because she was an alcoholic, she was compelled to continue drinking. When she stopped drinking, her alcoholism progressed. If she returned to drinking, the compulsion to drink would begin again.

The AA definition of alcoholism stresses self-definition. By the time the person wonders if he or she has a problem with drinking, the problem already exists. Nonalcoholics seldom if ever think about their drinking.

Comparing Definitions

Alcoholic Anonymous's operational definition of the alcoholic and alcoholism closely parallels those of the *DSM IV-TR* and the *ICD-10*. They concur that intoxication follows the ingestion of alcohol, which results in disturbances of levels of consciousness, cognition, perception, inhibitions, and other psychophysiological functions and responses. Sobering up occurs when drinking stops. Symptoms resolve over time. All agree that abuse of alcohol damages health. Likewise, the AA definition includes recognition of the development of a cluster of behavioral, cognitive, and physiological phenomena that develop after repeated substance abuse. These characteristics include a strong desire to continue use of the substance, increasing difficulties in controlling use of the substance, and continued use after recognition of its harmful consequences. AA recognizes the withdrawal state as being brought on by cessation of substance use and as occurring for a limited time. What AA calls *blackouts*, the *ICD-10* designates as *amnesic syndrome*, "a syndrome associated with chronic prominent impairment of recent and remote memory. Immediate recall is usually preserved and recent memory is characteristically more disturbed than remote memory. Disturbances of time sense and ordering of events are usually evident, as are difficulties in learning new material. Confabulation may be marked but is not invariably present. Other cognitive functions are usually relatively well preserved and amnesic defects are out of proportion to other disturbances."[33] Amnesic syndromes, or blackouts, can be experienced early or late in an alcoholic career.

AA's definition of alcoholism is an umbrella that includes all aspects of alcohol abuse. In AA the alcoholic is defined as "one whose life is made unmanageable to any degree by the use of alcohol." Although it lacks specificity, the definition precludes wasting time in the search for a "typical alcoholic" or "unitary alcoholism." The definition includes various patterns of alcoholic drinking. The practice content of AA logically includes examples of multiple types of alcoholism and recognition that as a phenomenon it is multifaceted. Above all, it is generally agreed that alcoholism is chronic, pervasive, and potentially fatal. It is characterized by initial tolerance to alcohol leading to unpredictability of reaction, physical dependence, and/or pathological organic change—all the direct logical consequences of drinking alcohol. It bears repeating that the AA mantra is that alcoholism can be arrested but can never be cured. It is defined, therefore, as a permanent condition of the alcoholic person, manifested along spiritual, mental, and physical lines.

The definition of alcoholism as a disease is ideologically integral to AA. It is important as a heuristic device and an explanatory mode. The medical accuracy of its use is not important to AA members; for them, its use explains the obsession with alcohol and compulsion to drink. This definition of alcoholism helps members identify with an acceptable explanation of their previous behavior. It promises change for the future. The binary nature of the AA definition brings the individual to a self-definition as an alcoholic. The disease "reasoning" is integral to much of the AA program. It creates a framework of definitions that allows for research and treatment. It makes compulsion and obsession, rather than choice, the common denominators of alcohol-related behavior. The model likewise provides a means of organizing past behaviors around an explanation that mitigates guilt based on new be- havior, unlike "moral choice" models. Further, the explanations inherent in the model are compatible with the program.

The Steps and their explications are always couched in terms of decisions about behavior, the adoption of that behavior, and the consequences of that adoption. The formal and the informal structures of AA work to change the array of possible responses to life events or perceptions of threat or reward. The drive to use alcohol as a solution, coping mechanism, or mood enhancer before that first drink is seen as having to do with the obsession portion of the definition and is seen as unique to the alcoholic. This obsession combined with the reaction to alcohol unique to the alcoholic brings about addiction. The assumption is that the alcoholic synthesizes alcohol differently from the nonalcoholic. That there is no scientific validity for the belief is of no impor- tance. It is common folk wisdom in AA and has the ring of truth to the mem- bers. Addictions so defined are treated with abstinence. It is also assumed that as sobriety and abstinence increases, alternative behaviors proliferate. As in all areas of life, abstinence involves ongoing choices that sustain it. Again, AA acts to provide a sociocultural context within which decisions are made and a new world emerges for the member. The references to choice in AA have to do with the decision to stop drinking: the decision to seek a different way of life, the decision to follow the dictates of the program, and the decision to experience the world differently. Choices always surround afflictions or states of being. AA emphasizes that the alcoholic's basic decision is whether or not to treat one's disease. As sobriety increases, so does the ability to make better choices about oneself and what conditions affect the experience of self.

3

ALCOHOL AND THE ALCOHOLIC

Alcoholics Anonymous defines alcoholism as having three aspects: physical, mental, and spiritual. Generally, the onset of alcoholism is slow. It is most recognizable in its physical and mental manifestations. Symptoms are initially subtle or infrequent in appearance. This gradual onset and growth allow for the individual's accommodation to the inconveniences and adjustments that alcohol abuse imposes in everyday life. As symptoms increase in severity, spiritual loss is reflected in the individual's demoralization and alienation. He or she loses fit and relevance.

"I'm a long-distance truck driver. Oh, I'm Greg, and I'm an alcoholic." The group laughs. Sometimes speakers are so eager to start that they forget to introduce themselves. Greg is about thirty years old. In his leather jacket and boots, he gives the impression that he can take care of himself. Even so, there is something gentle about his voice and smile. "Let's talk about change. It's been four years since I first came to AA. I didn't come on my own. The court sent me because of a drunken driving conviction. I don't know who was more upset—me or the cop. He stopped me because I was going too slowly. I told him I thought he was unreasonable to stop me for being careful. I told him that I had a lot to drink and I didn't want to have an accident. That was when he gave me a breath test. I went to jail for the night, every inch the victim.

"When my wife came to get me, I told her it was a mistake. She couldn't believe what happened. She said that she would know if I was a drunk. She had never seen me drunk. She meant really drunk. The truth was that I drank a little all the time. Jean was eighteen when we were married. I met her when I was twenty-one. We were together three months before we set up housekeeping. She had never known me when I didn't drink. The truth was that I had been drinking on a daily basis since I was twelve or thirteen. I never really got drunk, but I was never really sober. I didn't make a big deal about it. Some friends noticed some of what I did, but nobody knew about all of it. Everything I did was average. I got average grades. Teachers used to say I was polite but distant.

"My dad was a quiet guy also. Mom said I took after him. I spent a lot of time in my room drinking my dad's wine and beer. Dad made wine for himself and friends. He had oceans of it and didn't miss what I drank. I never gave any away. I drank it by myself. I started over-the-road driving right after high school. I liked it. I was alone on the road and made good money. What I'm getting at is that I was drunk all the time. No one knew me sober. It had been so long since I had been sober that even I couldn't remember what I had been like. God knows what I would have grown into if I hadn't used alcohol for fertilizer.

"I got older. I felt less and less connected to anyone or anything. It was nothing dramatic. I just felt empty and vaguely afraid. Jean couldn't get to me, and the kids were too young. I avoided them. I didn't drink any more; I just didn't drink less. I drank beer when I drove and when I was at home.

"When I got the DWI, I didn't care. I figured I'd get a fine and a lecture; no big deal. I hadn't hurt anyone, and my record was clean. The judge seemed sore as hell at me. My lawyer tried to be slick and to minimize the event. He talked about my clean record. As he was warming up to the subject, the judge told him to forget it and sit down. I was found guilty. The judge said he had had it with drunk drivers. I was to be his example. I got a year's probation, a large fine, and a restriction on my driving record. I was committed to an education program and AA four times a week. I was stunned. I howled that I couldn't do it. I worked. I had a family. It was my first time. The judge asked if I preferred to go to jail. His last words were, 'I hope you learn something.' He saved my life.

"For a while, all I could see was my resentment. What really scared me was that I couldn't drink. I couldn't imagine a day without drinking. Because the topic tonight is change, I'll just say that withdrawal was a bitch. I should have gone to a hospital, but I couldn't bring myself to go. I wasn't an alcoholic, I said. I just drank too much or too often. I did it all but I wasn't an alcoholic. Thanks to the judge, I went to AA four times a week, then five, and then seven. I never heard my story all at once but heard about feelings and events that I could identify with. The further away I got from my last drink, the more I marveled at what I felt. Every day I was experiencing emotions and feelings that were completely new. I didn't know what to do with them. I remember one night at home when I got mad at some minor thing. I think it was an insurance bill. I blew my top. Jean roared with laughter. She had never seen me 'lose my cool' before. I wasn't cool; I was numb. She liked it. I needed the experience. Later, I would learn more control. I had never known me sober; neither had anyone else. All of the fear, the general sickness, nervousness, and alienation I felt were the product of booze. I didn't know that because I was never without booze. Jean met a new guy. I was the same, but in a way I was different. My concerns included others. I got less selfish. I never thought of myself as selfish, but with a skin full of beer, I was. A lot of other things changed, to my surprise. I'm an outdoor person. I love to hunt and fish. Because I don't drink beer, I don't seem to enjoy the solitude of long-distance driving, but whenever I have an overnight, I go to a meeting. I always meet new friends there. Change for me has been slow and steady. In becoming sober, I'm a different guy. I didn't know what booze had done to me and how I had accommodated to it bit by bit. I have friends now, and they know what I'm like sober. Most don't know what I was like drinking. I hope the changes keep coming."

Because Greg began drinking early in his social development, his adjustments to alcohol took on the appearance of ordinary development. He never got the chance to see himself without booze. The development of Greg without alcohol may well provide surprises.

Many alcoholics describe the initial use of alcohol as helping shyness or feelings of inadequacy. For the alcoholic, the substance that relieves self-consciousness or gives confidence begins to impose conditions of its own. Drunkenness, forgetfulness, inappropriateness, and insensitivity to the needs or social cues of others are just a few of those impositions. There are good times with booze. There is a period in which it enhances things and creates the illusion of well-being. In many ways, alcoholics devastated by drinking continue to chase the good times they remember in early drinking. After a while, alcohol stops working.

Karen P. tells her story. "I was just starting college when I first began to drink wine. I was painfully shy in high school. I couldn't speak up in class. I didn't date. I just couldn't bring myself to do anything. I felt awkward and ugly. My grades were good, but I was definitely an oddball. My roommate in college knew how I felt. She was bouncy and bright. She wasn't particularly pretty, but she was popular—a real party girl. She said I was going to be her project.

"We fooled with makeup and clothes. I carried on conversations with boys who weren't there, for practice. Bonnie started to fix me up with boys. I tried, but I couldn't dance and couldn't talk. I was just so self-conscious. After a couple of months, Bonnie brought home a gallon bottle of red wine. She drank once in a while—a glass only. She had me drink a glass of the stuff before the next date. I was relaxed and talked. Everything had softness to it. When we went to the local hangout, I drank more wine. I knew I had found the solution. I flirted. In short, I was sensational.

"Over the years in college, I drank before and during dates and all the other important events. It relaxed me before tests. Sometimes it got me into trouble but not often. Once I fell asleep during a test, but I told the instructor that I was having my period. He was embarrassed and gave me a makeup. I thought then, and in some ways still think, that booze made me a complete person.

"After college, for some reason my drinking increased. I worked for a publishing house and was good at what I did. They liked me, but I drank more and more. By the time I turned thirty, I was sick at least half of the time from hangovers or being drunk. I didn't just drink to give me courage or the social graces. I drank all of the time. I was frightened in a vague kind of way. I had some physical symptoms—shaking hands and the sweats—but the psychological symptoms were the worst. All of my insecurities were back, but now I was full of self-loathing. Nothing went well. My job was more than I could handle. The more I drank the less I worked. I sat one night in my bathroom and drank almost a whole gallon of wine and couldn't get drunk. Booze just didn't work anymore. I drank for quite a while after that, trying to get the feeling back that I used to get when I drank. It never came back.

"After lunch one day I fell in my office. It took fifteen stitches to close the gash in my head. The doctor in the emergency room told the people who brought me that I was drunk. I wanted to die. I didn't. My boss offered me a choice—treatment or unemployment. I chose treatment. I have been sober for about three months. Some of my fears have abated. I still have all of the adjusting and growing up to do that booze prevented. I had problems when I drank, and I still have them. I think I can deal with them sober. I hope so."

For some, drinking is a social activity; for the alcoholic, never. *Social drinking* is a term devised by alcoholics. People without alcohol problems do not define themselves as drinkers of any sort. In the earlier stages of drinking, alcohol may serve the alcoholic as a kind of social lubricant. A few drinks gives previously unknown courage, and the wilted personality blossoms. After all, we live in a world that makes us all painfully self-conscious about our physical and verbal selves. Strict rules and standards apply, and for some people self-confidence is a fragile commodity requiring shoring up and reinforcement. Whatever the reason for the first drinking experience (almost inevitable in our society), the impact of alcohol on the system and personality of the alcoholic is immediate and oftentimes memorable. In AA it is frequently said that alcohol affects the alcoholic at initial intake differently than the nonalcoholic. While this may be after-the-event rationalization, there may be some truth to it. It is also congruent with the predominant AA view that alcoholism is a disease. In the early stages of drinking, alcoholics report that problems were solved and fears abated to one degree or another. Regardless of what inconveniences ensued, the early drinking experience is defined as positive. Alcohol for alcoholics initially carries an almost healing effect. It is the lubricant that smoothes their way in the world—until its effects become unpredictable.

As an activity, drinking is culturally defined as "adult," a sign of having arrived in a particular social place. Advertising placards exploit the image of the drinker as romantic and relate consuming alcohol to all forms of having fun. Indeed, it would seem that it is impossible to have any fun without alcohol. Among newly sober alcoholics, the most commonly expressed emotion is fear that "the good times are over; I'll never really laugh again." New social skills must be learned, and social interactions will evolve reflecting these new skills.

Regardless of the importance of alcohol in the social mix, the alcoholic does not drink for any of these reasons. The alcoholic drinks because he is compelled to. He is obsessed with alcohol and makes it the common denominator of his life. His addiction may manifest itself immediately or gradually, but regardless of the type of onset, the alcoholic is sentenced to dependency from the first drink. The culture facilitates access and makes drinking romantic and desirable, but, in my opinion, biological vulnerability in combination with cultural norms and imperatives make the alcoholic.

It is important not to confuse the trouble and social wreckage in the life of the alcoholic with reasons for drinking. The alcoholic does not drink because he has problems. He has problems because he drinks. After alcohol becomes part of the daily equation, the alcoholic creates his own problems and uses each in turn to rationalize drinking. He tends to think of alcohol as the glue that holds him together in a whirlwind of difficulties. From our point of view, most of his problems would disappear were he to stop drinking and begin to find his place in the normal run of things. Healing for the alcoholic demands more than abstinence. While healing begins with abstinence, it is only the beginning. Healing must address the threefold nature of the disease of alcoholism. It is one thing to stop drinking; it is quite another to stay stopped. Continuing sobriety demands growth and change. The Big Book, *Alcoholics Anonymous,* cautions that the same person unchanged will drink again.

The psychological and the physical are the most visible and measurable aspects of the disease. As such, they are the most amenable to traditional modes of medical, psychological, or psychiatric treatment. They also serve as the traditional benchmarks of recovery both to the alcoholic and those who are close to him. Later, I discuss just how the world of the alcoholic is pieced back together, but for now let us focus on the implications of the process of recovery in each of these areas.

The Physical Impact of Alcoholism

It is ironic that an early sign of alcoholism is the ability to consume and handle large quantities of alcohol. Countless AA stories start with "In the beginning, I could drink all night and take everyone else home." Nonetheless, the impact of sustained drinking on the body is enormous. Some of the damage is reversible, and some is not. Some damage is immediately apparent in the form of pain or other visible symptoms, such as passing blood through various orifices. Other damage makes itself apparent through loss of body functions (e.g., impotence, incontinence, or short-term memory loss). Another type of damage is manifested in shaking, inability to focus thoughts, senseless racing of thoughts, or simple formless mental meandering. Some of the most distressing symptoms, such as uncontrolled diarrhea and vomiting that frequently take up the morning hours, are more than familiar to the alcoholic whose problem has reached noticeable proportions.

A less recognizable, early physical sign of trouble ahead is the blackout. This state is not to be confused with sleep. The blackout is a short-term memory loss. In a blackout, the alcoholic frequently carries out complicated life processes and sometimes bizarre behaviors with no later memory of them.

This is most commonly expressed with such statements as "I don't remember how I got home last night"; "I don't know where I left my car"; "I don't recall that conversation." Whole evenings may be lost, and it is not unusual for an alcoholic who has experienced a blackout to call people and piece together the evening. These symptoms disappear and minor underlying pathologies quickly begin to heal when the alcoholic stops drinking. This very healing is dangerous. He feels better. He begins to rationalize that he could not have been that bad. He had the flu. Alcoholics love the flu. They have it all the time. The symptoms of the early stages of the flu are almost exactly those of the early stages of withdrawal from alcohol. Having the flu is more socially acceptable. It is easy to rationalize drinking at all hours of the day if you are doing it to alleviate flu symptoms.

The cycle of alcoholism does not seem to be that bad to the alcoholic. Life finally resolves itself into cycles of drinking and experiencing trouble of one kind or another or physical debilitation from excessive drinking. Being unable to predict what any amount of alcohol will do to the system may result in attempts at control. These attempts frequently result in short-term memory loss and other equally frightening symptoms of withdrawal. The body beginning the withdrawal process from alcohol is in pain. This is cured by the proverbial "hair of the dog that bit you." This is a daily cycle in the middle stages of the disease. Trouble is an ingredient in the mix. Many of the symptoms go unnoticed until they appear in combination. As symptoms become more florid, drinking becomes less controlled.

The alcoholic has turned a corner when he discovers that the majority of his symptoms can be alleviated by a drink in the morning. I doubt that anyone in this culture knows their body chemistry as well as the maintenance drinker who finds it necessary, in order to function, to keep a precise amount of alcohol in the bloodstream on a twenty-four-hour basis. He lives constantly on the edge of getting drunk or going into withdrawal. Consider the alcoholic cycle of life: drink until the symptoms become uncomfortable; stop for a while and let the body rest; resume drinking after the body has rested and starts to withdraw. For the alcoholic, any alternative is preferable to stopping drinking, and that most physical symptoms abate after a short period of time lends credence to the notion that damage is not permanent or serious.

These attitudes are reinforced by those persons closest to the alcoholic, who are frightened by his apparent alcoholism and his inability to manage his life. The family is frequently unwilling to stigmatize the individual alcoholic or themselves as the family of an alcoholic. The common phrase seems to be "Joe drinks too much but he isn't that bad." Families need to recognize the alcoholic in their midst. They need to confront and to believe in the possibility of arresting symptoms through abstinence.

The binge drinker is more difficult to diagnose. His periods of sobriety may vary greatly in length, as may his periods of drunkenness. The single fact that he appears to sober up after a bout with alcohol seems to support the idea that he can control his drinking. Of all alcoholics, the binge drinker seems least to fit the stereotype. The greater the length of time between binges, the less he fits the stereotype. As his binges get closer together, the closer he comes to approximating the stereotype. With great time gaps between bouts of drinking, the denial of alcoholism is easier to sustain. He is, nonetheless, an alcoholic. With the first drink, he cannot control his compulsion. His symptoms include all of the troubles and crazy behavior of the daily or weekend drinker. He may disappear for long periods of time and experience blackouts. When he is finally forced by biology or circumstance to stop drinking, his withdrawal, remorse, and isolation are as real a consequence as in the case of any other type of alcoholic.

This type of alcoholic is the most resistant to recovery and to the change demanded by that recovery process. Because of its arcane timing, his denial of his alcoholism receives enthusiastic support from friends and loved ones who find hope in the dry periods. Alcoholism is progressive and just as with other types, the periodic drunk experiences increasing severity of symptoms, increasing onset of occurrences, and less control and order in his life. His psychological deterioration continues at an increasing pace until, as is the case with all alcoholics, he reaches a bottom. The type and symptoms may vary, but the results of alcoholism are inevitable.

The Psychological Impact of Alcoholism

The psychological impact of alcohol on the alcoholic is dynamic. As people, we vary more psychologically than we do physically. We are more alike as biological entities than we are as psychological beings. Biologically, we share variations in a given gene pool and similarities imposed by species boundaries. Psychologically, the range of variations possible is limited only by the extremely broad range of environmental influences individuals can experience.

All aspects of socialization—that is, the process that makes us integrated, cognizant, acculturated beings—are mitigated by individual biological attributes and potentials. Consequently, the impact of alcohol in the individual varies more psychologically than it does physically. It is, therefore, more difficult to generalize about the psychological condition of the alcoholic or the impact of alcohol on that condition than it is to generalize about physical symptoms.

For the abuser, alcohol comes to be seen as the glue that holds the parts and pieces of self and world together. In the nonalcoholic, that glue may be drugs, or work, or some context of meaning. Some people conform. For some, life becomes the acting out of ritual until those rituals, devoid of meaning, become important in and of themselves. The literature of today's self-help psychology is sprinkled liberally with such terms as *workaholic* and *sleepaholic*. I have heard the term *sexaholic* used by a group advocating celibacy as the route to happiness and mental health. Such excesses, however, do not have their roots in biological vulnerability, as does alcoholism. A person's worldview, that is, the imperatives and prohibitions as well as what is valued and sought as the ultimate good, is shaped by some unifying influence. For the alcoholic, that unifying drive is alcohol.

It is not possible to isolate a particular "personality type" or group of personality characteristics that would enable us to separate the alcoholic from the nonalcoholic before the onset of the disease (frequently concomitant with the first drink). After the onset of the early, rewarding stages of alcoholism, elements of the personality become exaggerated. Because alcohol is a disinhibitor that dulls the wit as well as judgment, and all but eliminates social judgment, the alcoholic personality emerges as a product.

Alcoholic Anonymous's definition of the alcoholic is particularly useful. It defines the alcoholic as one whose life is made unmanageable to any degree by the use of alcohol. The famous "20 Questions" are useful. Their focus is on behavior and consequences. A single positive answer indicates a problem with alcohol. This definition makes no pretense. Its description is in everyday language and is meant to communicate rather than obviate.

20 QUESTIONS

Are You An Alcoholic?

To answer this question, ask yourself the following questions and answer them as honestly as you can:

1. Do you lose time from work due to drinking?
2. Is drinking making your home life unhappy?
3. Do you drink because you are shy with other people?
4. Is drinking affecting your reputation?
5. Have you ever felt remorse after drinking?
6. Have you gotten into financial difficulties as a result of drinking?
7. Do you turn to lower companions and an inferior environment when drinking?
8. Does your drinking make you careless of your family's welfare?
9. Has your ambition decreased since drinking?
10. Do you crave a drink at a definite time daily?
11. Do you want a drink the next morning?
12. Does drinking cause you to have difficulty in sleeping?
13. Has your efficiency decreased since drinking?
14. Is drinking jeopardizing your job or business?
15. Do you drink to escape from worries or trouble?
16. Do you drink alone?
17. Have you ever had a complete loss of memory as the result of drinking?
18. Has your physician ever treated you for drinking?
19. Do you drink to build up your self-confidence?
20. Have you ever been to a hospital or institution on account of drinking?

If you have answered YES to any one of the questions, there is a definite warning that you may be an alcoholic.

If you have answered YES to any two, the chances are that you are an alcoholic.

If you have answered YES to three or more, you are definitely an alcoholic.[1]

Later Stages of Alcoholism

Much of the literature addressing alcoholism focuses specifically on the later stages of the disease. This is particularly true with the literature of AA because it is directed at individuals who have reached a personal bottom and are either concerned about their drinking or seeking help in stopping drinking.

There are two identifiable patterns of influence. We are dealing with a personality that is as much the result of the consistent abuse of alcohol as any other factor considered in treatment or evaluation. We must take an inventory of the personality as it exists in the present and extrapolate to that period in the individual's life when alcohol was seldom used or did not appear to be a problem.

Within this framework, personality is an ever-changing, evolving presentation of self that is affected from moment to moment by the environment and, in a reciprocal sense, by the perception of that environment. Think of the personality as a bit of onion that is constantly being peeled. With each peeling (presentation of self), a new and different yet similar layer is shown. The pre-alcohol personality will provide a benchmark against which the alcohol-influenced presentation of personality may be judged. Alcohol produces pathologies in the personality, altering awareness and mitigating against empathy.

In the AA model, the biologically rooted compulsion to drink, combined with alcohol, will affect certain aspects of personality more than others. Alcohol generates extremes. Change occurs when alcohol is removed from the life of the alcoholic. Extremes are reduced as predictability and reason return. Alcoholics must learn to live sober. This process is as foreign to them as the process of maintaining a slightly drunken edge, twenty-four hours a day, is to nonalcoholics. They must learn to cope with new emotions not blunted by alcohol. They must learn to deal with perceptions not fogged by alcohol. It is AA's contention that, for alcoholics to stop drinking and stay stopped, they need a way of life that provides an ethical, moral, and functional basis for living sober. They need a social structure that supports a sober life. For this reason, the program initially takes up a lot of time and appears to be all inclusive in its scope and its mandates for change. Paradoxically, the result is that people change dramatically and remain essentially themselves.

His Majesty the Infant Rules the World

The AA description of the alcoholic is neither subtle nor academic. The thrust of its specification is not so much diagnostic as utilitarian and instructive of remedial need. In general, it describes alcoholics as being many and varied. Even so, they have certain characteristics in common. The first of these characteristics is an overwhelming concern with self. That is, they tend to relate to events in the lives of others only as those events affect them. For example, the death of a parent or friend is viewed not in terms of the impact of that death on others but in terms of what inconveniences, difficulties, or loss the death causes the alcoholic.

You might say that the individual prefaces his life with "I." He is an example of self-will run riot. The need to control others is evident. He wants to run the show. He is unhappy with the scenario as written and views that as the fault of others. "If only other people would do what I want them to do," or "treat me properly," or "would do what I think they should do," then, finally, "everything would be all right." He is self-seeking and selfish in the extreme. Even in his apparent service to others there is an element of self-seeking in terms of benefits and self-aggrandizement. His acts are never selfless. His interactions are characteristically dishonest.

As his disease progresses, it is as if he lies when the truth would serve better. It is almost as if he is lying to keep in practice. He is dishonest with himself about his disease and with others who are concerned about him. The impact of his increasing dependence on alcohol forces an increasingly dishonest lifestyle. Given this configuration of personality, it is not surprising that the alcoholic is also full of self-pity and anger at self and others. He deludes himself with regard to his behavior and his relationships with others. He is characteristically a grudge-holder and full of resentment.

As he bounces from one dramatic event or crisis to another, these resentments grow and fester. It is part of his self-delusion that he is not responsible for anything that happens to him. He is the perpetual victim. He is the classic "injustice collector." His motto could be, "Never forget and never give an inch." In the literature of AA, the alcoholic is described as a whirlwind roaring through the lives of others. Only sobriety can calm the winds and prevent future damage. It is a dramatic characterization, but it provides characteristics for identification.

In an address delivered at the Ninety-ninth Annual Meeting of the American Psychiatric Association in Dearborn, Michigan, in 1943, Dr. Harry M. Tiebout, a professional associated with the early development of Alcoholics Anonymous, offered a similar, albeit more diagnostically oriented, set of alcoholic personality characteristics. He suggested that the alcoholic was a "narcissistic, egocentric [person], dominated by feelings of importance, intent on maintaining, at all cost, his inner integrity." He went on to say that, while these characteristics can be found in varying degrees in persons both normal and seeking help, they appear "in a relatively pure culture in alcoholic after alcoholic. The alcoholic brooks no control from man or God. He, the alcoholic, is, and must be, master of his destiny. He will fight to the end to preserve that position."[2]

It is irrelevant whether these personality characteristics are the product or by-product of the compulsion to drink or if they were present in the individual as personality penchants before the individual drank. What is important is that these characteristics appear to be uniformly found in alcoholics seeking help. Regardless of what basic ingredients the alcoholic brings to the development of his own personality, the impact of alcohol creates interesting and devastating aberrations. The alcoholic experiences an increasingly shrinking world.

Tiebout pinpointed such specific problems as aggression, feelings of being at odds with the world, and negativity. Change in this pessimistic picture, according to Dr. Tiebout, can be brought about by involvement with Alcoholics Anonymous. "Until any change is linked with the mind and the intellect, the cure is considered suspect." His comments seem as germane today as they were in 1943.

Returning to the AA model, the alcoholic's loss of priorities begins with the intake of alcohol. All things in life are second to the compulsion to drink. The person is dominated by the obsession with alcohol. What appears to be voluntary drinking is in reality compulsive behavior.

A young woman, Janet R., told of beginning to drink in her early teens. At the time she was a good student and had no real difficulty with friends or family. She was evidently sensitive to alcohol because she drank constantly. She failed in school, and her old friends were forgotten. Because she drank daily, she chose friends in school who had similar interests. Her relationship with her family deteriorated. Concerned with her drinking and resultant wildness and depression, her family had her committed to a mental institution. Her alcoholism had isolated her and depressed her to the brink of suicide. She couldn't articulate what was wrong. Her drinking was considered a symptom of pathology rather than the cause of one.

She was given shock therapy. After several sessions, Janet later remembered, a doctor asked: "Do you know who you are?" "No." "Do you know where you are?" "No." "Do you know who I am?" "No." "Do you know what has happened to you?" "No." "Can we do anything for you?" Janet recalled asking for a drink. Throughout her hospitalization and various therapies, no one suggested that her drinking had anything to do with her problems. While drinking she found it difficult to separate her feelings from those experienced in the hospital where she was heavily sedated. After a number of attempts at therapy, she finally found a therapist who asked her how much she drank. Unlike most alcoholics in therapy, she told the truth. The therapist said he thought that the drinking was her problem and suggested AA. As she spoke, Janet was celebrating eight years of sobriety. Her symptoms had disappeared with the alcohol.

The obsession to drink seems to have a life of its own. It is at the core of the alcoholic identity. For the alcoholic, booze is mother's milk. Janet's story illustrates that alcohol can produce symptoms not unlike mental illness. The confusion begins when alcohol is seen as the symptom of pathology rather than the cause of it. In these cases, abstinence is the medicine best prescribed. Studies have indicated that there is a link between alcoholism and affective disorders. At times, the symptoms appear identical. There also appears to be a link between alcoholism and certain eating disorders. As tempting as speculation is, we leave these discoveries to the further unraveling of the DNA puzzle.

Denial

Dixon B. began drinking while in high school. "I was shy and a few beers made everything easy. It was easier to meet girls, and I made a lot of friends. Alcohol was not a problem. I liked to drink, but I didn't feel I had to. A pattern was established, however. Beer became a part of every social occasion. When I started my career I had long since forgotten that I had ever been shy. I drank beer all of the time, but I still didn't associate it with trouble. I got married, had kids, and drank more and more beer. I drank at work during lunch and around two o'clock. I owned the place. Why not? I went right home after work, ate, drank beer, watched TV, and went to sleep. My wife, Doris, and I used to do things together. We didn't anymore. I blamed the kids. It was the beer.

"As time passed I was less and less available for outside activities. Doris and I fought a lot; mostly about my drinking. One day I woke up and found myself all alone. The only time I left the house was to go to work. At work I did pretty much what I did at home. Doris had developed a set of friends and activities on her own. I was relieved when she went out. I could drink without her hearing everything. Finally, I stopped going to work. My living room had become my world. I drank my way into detox. Now I don't drink at all. My world includes a lot more now. I've had to learn how to live sober. I can't believe I ever lived like that. I started to drink to help me be social and expand my world. I ended up in my own house all alone. It's easier to be sober."

The alcoholic's world shrinks as the focus on alcohol and drinking grows. As the dependence on alcohol increases, the dependence on others for social commerce decreases. He finds himself avoiding friends and family alike. He does this because they represent the pointing finger of guilt. They generate feelings of frustration and guilt and, by their presence, act as a kind of externalized conscience. As the alcoholic's dependence on drink increases, alcohol increasingly structures his life. The combination of this obsession and physical dependence orders his day in terms of what he will drink, when he will drink, and how much he will drink. His dual concerns include the invention of ways to hide his drinking and a need to secure an adequate supply of alcohol. He must also find a way of handling contact with the nonalcoholic world. He must protect his job or profession by any means. Even the weekend or binge drinker has these needs, and job performance will be affected by his drinking patterns.

The facade of normalcy for the drinker can be shored up only by lying about money, about physical whereabouts, about activities, and about friendships. The basic elements in a marriage such as predictability, fidelity, and trust are quickly eroded. All this juggling takes a lot of fancy footwork and deception. The alcoholic, however, protects his need for alcohol from discovery. It is his assumption that he drinks because he has troubles. He sees alcohol as the only thing that is helping him get from day to day. Without it, he would drown in a sea of difficulties. Of course, he believes these troubles have their origins outside of him.

The illusion that alcohol is a positive element in an otherwise negative world is probably the most devastating aspect of the disease of alcoholism. AA wisdom suggests that the alcoholic's belief that he can control his drinking or learn how to drink like "normal" people do may well lead him to insanity or death. As dramatic as that sounds, the alcoholic is engaged in a life-and-death struggle. Alcoholism invariably leads to one of two conclusions. The first is insanity. The second, death, may occur through organ

failure, accident, or suicide. Alcoholics often choose suicide as an alternative
to living a life of deception, spiritual and emotional poverty, and isolation.
Where alcoholism and depression coexist, the impact of alcohol exacerbates
the depression and is particularly dangerous.

More subtle symptoms occur outside of the normal interactive framework
of the alcoholic. One of the more devastating later-stage symptoms is the onset of unreasonable fears or what the individual might perceive as undifferen-
tiated, free-floating anxiety. Many fears appear to be grounded in perceptions
of personal vulnerability. Alcohol-related fears may include an inability to get
in and out of elevators; fear of driving, bridges, telephones, or the mail; or just
a general fear of everything. These fears become acute at night. Alcoholics do
not sleep as deeply or as restfully as nonalcoholics. Sleep apnea is common.
In the late stages of alcoholism, the individual frequently wakes up two or
three times a night with the body demanding a drink. Noises in the house,
noises outside of the house, and fears of intrusions are all exaggerated and
preclude sleep.

Sober alcoholics report disposing of mattresses on which the outlines of
their bodies are etched in sweat. Sweat and chills frequently accompany attempts to sleep. Imagine lying in a bed, sweating profusely, feeling alternately
hot and cold, unable to sleep, full of fear, and conjuring up all manner of
demons while ruminating about the futility of life and the inability to control
one's destiny. Being an alcoholic who drinks is not easy. Fears are accurate
predictions of the future. Given the nature of the alcoholic's lifestyle, obligations are seldom met on time, credit is abused, bad checks are written, and
employers are frequently in search of lost employees. In such circumstances,
fear of the future is understandable.

Generally, active alcoholics do not like themselves much. By the time they
talk to anyone about their drinking problem, they have already lost control
over central elements in their lives and cannot seem to regain it. At this point
in the progression of their disease, they have usually tried to stop drinking
with varying degrees of success. They have returned to drinking and found
that their disease and their dependence on alcohol have progressed even during dry periods. "How did I end up here again?" "Why do these things happen to me all the time?"

We must keep in mind that alcoholics phrase these questions in terms of
what is being done to them. Consequently, the denial and defenses stay intact.
In their minds, their problem is not alcohol; they have other problems. They

believe they can control alcohol, and this illusion prevents them from putting their lives back together. Bosses don't understand, friends don't understand, and the alcoholics themselves don't understand. However, they cannot stop drinking and fear what will happen if they do. They reason that if they had fewer problems they would drink less.

Alcoholism and Spirituality

The impact of alcohol on the alcoholic is physically and psychologically devastating. The impact of the disease on the spirit is perhaps the most elusive and yet the most crucial to understand. The spiritual life is seldom discussed in our daily lives. Little wonder that we are confused or even put off by any consideration of a lifestyle or commitment that has at its base spiritual considerations. Spirituality in this context is more than belief in mystery or things unexplained in the language of demonstration and science. It is more than belief in a God or, for that matter, any systems based on obligation, ritual, and eventual reward. It is more than belief in the magical or miraculous explanation of things or events that seem to contradict the order, process, or scientific explanation of things as we understand them.

Spirituality is in our relationship to others. It is sensitivity to social and psychological fit and awareness of the place of others. It is the sense of being central in a stream of consciousness that defines an ethical base. For the alcoholic, as with other people, the loss of the spiritual life (which we see as being derived from interaction with others in common enterprise) is gradual and difficult to define. Its loss is the origin of the often-described feeling of anxious despair, of groundless fear and isolation so often shared by thousands of alcoholics in thousands of AA meetings over the world. Not only does the spirit erode, it can all but cease to be. It can cease to evolve with age and the life experiences that normally temper and develop it. Spirituality is relational. It involves interaction with others and with the world of ideas and things. Some seem to manage relations with others and the rules of life easily, naturally. Others seem to swim upstream all of their lives. Some of these differences in style lie in the differences in biological makeup that distinguish us one from the other.

All that impinges on us physically or psychologically is integrated through unique filters that themselves are the result of socialization. All people react to learning in varying degrees and adapt within genetic limits. In growing up we develop feelings about ourselves and about others that structure new interactions. Others react to us on the basis of how they perceive our "fit" in the world of ideas and the appropriateness of our behavior. A significant part of our self-image depends on how others react to us. How real are we to others? We are a delicate mix—actor and audience, a mechanism that requires constant momentum in the areas of attitude and social posture. The person who negotiates life comfortably with a positive self-image has a sense of correctness about himself. His personality and self are a process integrated with the interactional world and the world of meanings around him.

For the drinking alcoholic, such growth and reciprocal sensitivity cannot exist. The spirit does not grow. It is reduced by the isolation and negative psychological state that accompanies the use of alcohol. Self-image is most profoundly affected. Just as others in the culture reject alcoholism, the alcoholic rejects himself, his inability to manage his life and his helplessness. In short, the alcoholic has lost his "fit" with the world of meaning. He has made his validity as a person dependent on things and meanings that are external to him.

The spiritual is more elusive to define and to map than other elements that make up the human condition. That it is diminished, compromised, and even extinguished by alcoholism is perhaps obvious only to the alcoholic. We have few ways to measure the loss of the spiritual life, and, as is the case with so many other aspects of alcoholism, the loss is so gradual as to be barely perceptible. Symptoms of this loss, however, manifest themselves with increasing intensity and frequency as the disease of alcoholism runs its inevitable course.

At an Al-Anon meeting held in a large old church basement in the center city area, Violet P. talked about spirituality. She didn't drink, but her husband did until about a year ago. He's in AA; she attends Al-Anon. As she puts it, the kids just sit around and watch the changes. Vi attended Al-Anon meetings for three years before her husband finally threw in the towel. She is a composed woman with a strong voice.

"Well, you have heard it before, but I either had to throw him out or learn how to live with what was going on in my life. Tony was drinking all the time, and the only time we saw him was when he came home to fight or sleep. Sometimes he felt guilty, and we would talk, and he would try to slow down or promise to manage, but he couldn't. I didn't know that alcoholism was a family disease. I thought that it was Tony's problem. I was dependent on him financially, and with three small children I felt helpless.

"Tony ran his own business, a gas station and garage. He was open eighteen hours a day and was always in and out. The more he stormed and complained about the way I ran the house and the kids, the more I began to feel responsible. At the end, he had me believing that I was responsible for all of the trouble. I didn't understand why he came or went, or why he complained that I 'never cooked shit for dinner!' I cooked for him all the time. When I did cook, he didn't like it. I don't know if it's true or not—Tony says it isn't—but one of his friends said that at the station one night, Tony said, 'I'm going to go home and pitch a bitch if dinner ain't on the table.' 'What if it's ready?' He said, 'Not going to eat it.'

"I guess the point is that I couldn't do anything right. I couldn't support myself and the kids. I was a lousy wife and a lousy mother. I was fat. I was stupid. I was a nag. I bitched about Tony's drinking all the time. The more I complained and begged him to stop, the more he said I was the problem. None of the kids were doing well in school. They were frightened to death of their father. Even today they don't trust him.

"It all seemed so normal. I mean it was so gradual. Tony started drinking at home. The kids spent more and more time outside. I dropped what few friends I had outside of the home. I stopped having my hair done. I stopped shopping for new clothes. The house became my world, and I slopped around in shapeless housecoats all day. It was gradual, but in about four years I had become what Tony called me. I watched the soaps and put my head in neutral. Tony and I stopped having a physical relationship around that time.

"A year or so later, he revived our physical relationship. He started slapping me when I talked back to him. Still, I felt I needed him. I loved him. After he beat me up, he was always so sweet. It never lasted long. He would drink; I would cry and eat. A couple of more years went by. Thank God the business almost ran itself. Tony's manager encouraged him to stay at home more and more. When Tony broke up the furniture, I cleaned it up. When he got sick all over the house, I cleaned it up. When I added myself up, I got zero.

"The kids ignored me and were in trouble at school. I just couldn't get motivated enough to do anything. I felt empty, hollow. I couldn't see the point in anything. I felt responsible and guilty. I still felt a certain kind of identification with Tony. The slapping around was a regular ritual in which my identity and guilt were confirmed, and Tony's insane drive to control was satisfied. As Tony slipped more and more into alcoholic drinking and crazy behavior, I began to lose myself. Tony's alcoholism terrorized the kids and created problems that we are still trying to deal with. My maladies were of the spirit. I lost myself somewhere along the way.

"One afternoon, during a break in a television program, I saw an ad for Al-Anon. It was short but gave a phone number. I called and went to a meeting later that week. It took a while, but I began to identify with the women I heard. Each of them felt responsible and diminished by the way they lived. I heard answers. From the moment I separated myself from the consequence of Tony's drinking, I began to feel better. It took a long time (about six months), but I began to do things for myself. I stopped confronting Tony, but I also stopped catering to him. The first night I tried to put my new philosophy into action, I was frightened but determined. Tony came home drunk. He fell on the porch and rolled half onto the lawn. I left him there for the neighbors in the morning.

"I put the house on a regular meal schedule and kept it clean and neat. I visited school and started to work with the kids. Throughout this, Tony raised hell. The first time he slapped me, I called the cops. He got tough with them. They put him up for the night. I let him come home, but I told him that if he ever slapped me again I would have him arrested. He slugged me about three months later. I had him arrested and pressed the charge. He moved out and refused to give me any money. I embarrassed him to the point where he paid the bills. I even took money out of the cash register. A kind of magic happened. I learned that I could say no and make it stick.

"Tony came home. He kept on drinking, and I didn't nag him about it. I didn't buy his booze. I didn't serve it to him. If he missed a meal, he could fend for himself. I tried to understand him. I wanted him to get well, but I couldn't do it for him. I took responsibility for myself and managed the house. Gradually, I began to feel better about me. I turned things I couldn't control over to my higher power. I felt less frustrated. I trusted the Al-Anon program. After a while, I took a volunteer job at the state hospital. I'm there three days a week. If I ever have to support myself, I think I could now. I do Tony's books at the station. The more I sorted myself out, the better I felt about me.

"It's been a long time and a hard time. I feel in step with the world again. The more I asserted myself, the more I felt I had rights. I stopped apologizing for being around. I think I went too far the other way. I got bossy with the kids and with Tony. That stopped when I started to work on my resentments. Tony's straight now, but things are strained between us. I am not certain that we're going to make it. I am certain, however, that alcoholism caused me to lose myself. Meanings in life ceased to exist for me. I think of it now as the death of my interior. I'm staying close to Al-Anon."

Violet's story is not unique. What is important for us to understand, however, is the systematic loss of her feelings of self-worth and purpose. Her inability to come to grips with alcoholism as a family disease caused a lot of problems. Every member of a family is affected by the alcoholism of any single member. Violet began to find herself when she related alcohol to her spiritual malady. When she got herself in order, stopped trying to control her husband's drinking, and got over her resentments, she found her spiritual anchors again. What put Violet on the track of dealing effectively with her feelings of loss, low self-worth, fear, and helplessness was action. She did not theorize or intellectualize her way to spiritual growth and awareness. On a day-to-day basis she acted on faith. She came to believe that a life based on ethical and moral principles could restore her to spiritual and mental health, and she acted on those principles.

Later, at an AA meeting, Tony told his story. Violet figured prominently. "I got off the down elevator early in my drinking career. Vi's getting to Al-Anon had something to do with it. When she stopped fighting and complaining, I started feeling guilty. When she had me arrested, I realized what I had done and what I had become. I never intended to slap my wife around. It was as if we just slipped into it. I had to control her, and I thought she needed or wanted to be controlled.

"I was desperate all of the time, and I couldn't lose the feeling of helplessness. My emotions were always on the surface, and I exploded with little provocation. When I tried to take care of business, I made a mess of it. I couldn't stand myself, and I couldn't stand her. I hated my life but wouldn't do anything to change it. The truth was I didn't know what I wanted or what was wrong. When I thought about changing things, I thought of everything but giving up booze. The more Vi screamed about it, the less I thought it was the root of my problems. Nothing scared me as much as the thought of stopping drinking. It was the only thing that helped.

"I drank for a couple of years after Vi got help in Al-Anon. She became a different person. She came on like she was the strong one. She had the answers. I couldn't control her, and now I couldn't even control myself. Drinking wasn't fun anymore, but I kept it up. One drunken afternoon, I called AA. I wanted to tell them to get the hell out of my life. I had never been to a meeting.

The guy I talked to said he understood what was going on with me. I agreed to have someone come over and talk. Barry H. found me half drunk and feeling sorry for myself. Instead of lecturing me, he told me about himself and how it felt at the time he decided that he had had enough. We went to a 5:30 meeting.

"I drank after that, but I got the message. Vi encouraged me but didn't insist or nag. I used to complain about her going to meetings. I started going to meetings too. AA has brought about a lot of changes in me, but I haven't been sober long enough to take it for granted. One day at a time, I'm putting my life back together. The fears have left me. I'm going to keep living on a day-to-day basis. I'm sure things are going to work out the way they should be."

Not all alcoholic husbands slap their wives around. The need to control has many faces. Not all wives of alcoholics go to Al-Anon. Alcoholics do, however, share a loss of spirit, and their families experience a common loss. The spiritual condition of the individual is not the common currency of everyday conversation. In fact, outside of a few special groups, a sure way to be considered to be a little bit out of whack is to discuss the spiritual life and to relate it to anything real or relevant in the world.

Consider the plight of the alcoholic in such a milieu; his world shrinks and his mind and reality contact are so eroded by booze that his social and spiritual isolation is all but complete. As his world becomes more and more focused on him and his compulsion to drink dominates, significant elements of identity and security become lost. Usually, legal and financial crises attend the later stages of the disease as calamity follows calamity and isolation increases. Feelings of self-worth disappear. Traditional values and social anchors are eroded by the process of drinking. Their loss becomes a reason to drink. The circle is complete. The alcoholic insists that he drinks because he has problems. In truth it is that the alcoholic drinks, and so he has problems. In addition, he exists in a culture that does not recognize the need for a spiritual "fit," nor does it provide institutionalized ways to mend the troubled spirit.

What Do We Believe about the Alcoholic?

Our stereotype of the alcoholic is etched in the literature and films of the last several decades. The stereotype is most frequently male and ranges from the benign, elfin, Irish drunk, to the confused and hopeless drunk in the movie

The Lost Weekend. From time to time, a depiction includes hope for recovery, as recently seen in the film *Days of Wine and Roses.* Overall, the stereotype of the alcoholic is that of a person with profligate habits and a weak will. The alcoholic is viewed as the author of his own ills, who has his own cure at his fingertips if only he could "take hold of himself" and stop that damn drinking. It is the stigmatized image of the alcoholic that makes the disease of alcoholism such a shame. Common understanding has it that the individual does not have an affliction; he has a condition that he has brought about by himself and could control, if only he would. The fact that he doesn't control his drinking is proof of his lack of worth, his lack of willpower, his inability to take care of himself, and his lack of concern for those around him. The question "Why do you do this when you know what will happen to you?" goes unanswered, but the socially interpreted answer is implicit in the question itself. The question assumes that the alcoholic has control over his drinking. Probably the most pernicious aspect of the stereotype of the alcoholic is that he believes it himself. Alcoholism is not something that requires treatment; rather, it is something that needs hiding and, most importantly, denying.

Because he believes his drinking is the result of poor willpower or bad judgment, the alcoholic believes he can stop or control drinking by an act of will. He can do it himself. Sharing his problem will label him publicly as a weakling. As long as the alcoholic sees his drinking problem as the result of personal failing rather than a biological condition combined with socialization, he will seek a solution within himself. The culture tells him the solution is there inside of him. As long as the solution is sought individually and seen as the exercise of willpower or self-control, failure is all but inevitable. Paradoxically, the complimentary stereotype to this version of the alcoholic is that of the Bowery bum or the derelict. The derelict is the quintessential alcoholic. In the eyes of many, he is the alcoholic. It's for this reason that alcoholics are often told by persons closest to them that they aren't that bad, that their only problem is that they drink a little too much. They are not alcoholics. Things are what we believe them to be. The resolution of alcohol-related problems for alcoholics lies outside of themselves; sobriety requires a structured support system that addresses the complexity of the problem.

Discussion of the spiritual elements in our lives must focus on the beliefs that constitute our worldview. This may include belief in traditional forms of God, complete with heaven and hell, good and bad, reward and punishment, and a lifetime of behavior being sorted out at some time in the future. Or our worldview may not include belief in these things. If it doesn't, how does the individual relate to the legitimacy of moral rules or societal mandates? What constitutes authority? What is our direction in the dance of mankind?

The concern here is how each of us perceives his or her "fit" in the world's general operations. Many of the problems that people have in their day-to-day lives can be labeled psychological or called crises of the spirit or, at the very least, spiritual in nature. In short, how people perceive themselves in the world, their sense of worth, their perceptions of how others see and value them, their views, their belief in their own potential and its realization, their chance of achievement and how they perceive the roles of others in that process, is spiritual in nature and based on belief rather than experience or facts. We create much of our reality, and by acting as if it were so, we make it so. Our beliefs create self-fulfilling prophecies in our lives. This is certainly true in the case of the alcoholic. Remove the alcohol from the equation, and the world of the alcoholic changes. It becomes more related to the main themes of the culture.

The alcoholic has lost his "fit" in the culture. He has lost touch with the essence of his world. Because of his alcoholism, he cannot find in the culture answers to the fundamental existential questions of self-direction, action, morality, and purpose. His alcoholism is an unshareable problem. The alcoholic's isolation, grandiosity, skewed perceptions of relationships in the world and his role in it, coupled with unreasoning fears and deteriorating physical condition, ruin his chances of participating in satisfying or meaningful activities in the culture.

Additionally, the present-day American culture, with its focus on technology and progress, does not offer the integration of the spiritual life with the daily physical activities of life. If anything, we seem all but embarrassed at the mention or inclusion of spirituality, even when divorced from its traditional religious trappings, in any of our daily activities. It is almost as if ethical and moral prescriptions are interpreted as rules to be applied where convenient, rather than as blocks on which to build a satisfying life.

While other relationships are tenuous or of short duration, the alcoholic's relationship to booze, combined with its devastating psychical impact and the biologically rooted compulsion to drink, remains constant. The erosion and skewing of his or her worldview is equally constant. "He could stop if he really wanted to." This erroneous set of beliefs compounds the alcoholic's drinking problem and precludes a solution to it. Continued drinking exacerbates feelings of failure with resultant negative self-image. The culture tells the alcoholic that he has a problem he must solve himself. The alcoholic believes this. He, therefore, seeks solution in self-discipline, in moderation, in the substitution of other drugs or similar attempts.

Because the person is attempting to solve the problem of alcoholism alone, he or she is doomed to failure. He seeks therapy on the basis of defining his need to drink as being rooted in some psychological pathology, traceable to an early trauma, to how he was reared, to his relationship with his parents, or similar reasons. Until he understands that his alcoholism is rooted in his biology and not in his psyche, he is doomed to fail. His existential condition in many ways can be defined as a symptom of his biological vulnerability. Any attempt to arrest alcoholism must deal with its physical, psychological, and spiritual aspects. The only alternative is abstinence.

4

GETTING SOBER

The alcoholic has "lost his fit." He has lost his place in the social and occupational systems that anchor us all in the culture. The experience is one of existential alienation. He experiences spiritual loss that is manifested in every aspect of his interior life and interactions with other people. He experiences physical and psychological problems. He can neither stop drinking nor continue on his life path. Normal touchstones of identity are seriously eroded or absent. He has come undone and is out of control. Getting sober and staying sober are his only viable options.

The process of getting sober and staying sober is so simple, and so mechanically uncomplicated, that for the alcoholic, it is easy to overlook or misunderstand. It is also probably the hardest thing in this world for the alcoholic to do. A friend said, "It's like tiger stew. It's simple; it's only hard at the beginning to catch the tiger." Getting sober is like that: the first part is hard to do, and all the rest depends on it.

Recognition: The Bottom

Is the alcoholic ready to change? Has he or she hit bottom or at least found some compelling reason to get sober? In simplest terms, the bottom is the point at which the alcoholic knows he can go no further. Whatever else happens in his life, he knows that he has to stop drinking. In all probability, he does not know what will be left when the alcohol is gone, but whatever it is will be better than now. Any change can only be an improvement.

Willingness to change may be fleeting. The awareness of alcohol as the evil in his life may not last long. The resolve to quit drinking "forever" may evaporate after the first physical symptoms disappear or the precipitating crisis is over. However, once the connection is made between the chaos, the despair, and alcohol, a bottom is at hand. Drinking alcoholics are generally not aware of the connection between their drinking and the troubles in their lives. The majority are either afraid to admit the connection or deny it by defining alcohol as the only thing that enables them to deal with the crisis in their lives. Usually, by the time the alcoholic has reached this point, he had tried unsuccessfully to control or stop his drinking. He may not recognize his compulsion to drink, but he does know that he is drinking when he does not want to. Alcohol is taking him places he does not want to go and making him do things he does not want to do. At the very least, he is a bundle of confused and conflicted emotions. He is willing to do anything to continue drinking and yet despises his inability to stop. At this point, most alcoholics really do not want to stop drinking, but they do not want to continue either. Alcohol's effect has, in most instances, become unpredictable. A small amount of alcohol may get the individual drunk, whereas at other times he will be able to consume enormous amounts with no apparent effect. His body simply does not metabolize in a regular, predictable way. If this is not the most common single element that triggers a perception of bottom in the alcoholic, it is one of the most frequently cited.

In some cases, the events that precipitate a bottom are catastrophic: driving while under the influence, being arrested and jailed for an alcohol-related event, or being fired from a treasured job. The alcoholic may be left by spouse and children or thrown out of the house by parents. He may suffer physical collapse, delirium tremens, hospitalization for alcoholism, withdrawal while in an alcoholic rehabilitation program, or the like. Social and economic circumstances can affect the timing and the nature of a bottom. As wisdom has it, the elevator goes down a lot of floors; you can get off at any level.

The amount of residual damage from drinking varies from individual to individual. The critical factor seems to be individual tolerances and perception of severity. Social supports such as family and friends may help or hinder self-awareness. Friends or family who make excuses for the drinker enable the abusive patterns to continue. Old wisdom had it that intervention needed to await the final disaster, that is, the end of the road or the bottom. More modern thinking suggests that intervention can occur at almost any stage of the descent. The key to effectiveness is consequences. The family that confronts a member, forcing him or her to see the impact of drinking on oneself and family, and is willing to impose consequences can create a bottom. Results from such interventions may not be immediately apparent but always serve to foster awareness. Incidentally, when they are a surprise to the alcoholic, such interventions also generate confrontation and anger. Depending on the individual, a number of interventions and consequences may be required. The earlier the intervention, the more likely the residual damages from alcoholism can be minimized.

A bottom may also be precipitated by an accumulation of feelings of despair and anxiety culminating finally in the alcoholic's feeling that he is existentially near death and devoid of hope. Regardless of what precipitates the bottom for the individual alcoholic, the psychological state is more important than the physical props or circumstances surrounding the occurrence. In a sense, despair is despair, regardless of what precipitates it. We are all different. It is little wonder that the conditions of initial surrender differ. Bottoms, therefore, vary from alcoholic to alcoholic. Alcoholism is a progressive disease. As the alcoholic progresses in his drinking, each valley will be deeper and each crisis more serious. The actual event precipitating surrender to treatment, however, may not be the most serious consequence of drinking. It will simply be the last incident. It may be the final drop that tips the scale.

Just as many drinking patterns are affected by social class, variables such as financial status and education affect bottoms. In AA, one hears of high-bottom drunks and low-bottom drunks. The thrust of the distinction is to designate how closely the alcoholic approaches the derelict stereotype when he arrives at the doors of AA asking for help. More colorfully put, "Yale or jail, it doesn't matter where you come from. What matters is where you are." Personal loss as a result of alcoholism is variously defined. The wealthy may have more material things and more prestigious jobs to lose, but the loss of everything—family, home, and job—is as serious to a blue-collar worker as to a bank president. Shame, guilt, and bitterness know no social boundaries. Having an abundance of money can help forestall the consequences of drunkenness, but, as they say at AA, "eventually for all of us the chickens come home to roost."

Ralph E. discussed his bottom at a meeting he chaired. His subject was resolution and surrender, and on this particular evening he wanted to talk about what brought him to AA. "The first time I came to AA, I did not arrive humble, with hat in hand. I called AA and went to my first meeting because I was in a lot of pain and couldn't stop drinking. In all honesty, I don't think

I wanted to stop drinking. I wanted to stop hurting and above all I wanted to learn how to drink. I thought that if I could limit my binging to a few days during the month, the rest of my life would be manageable.

"My experience with alcohol had paralleled all of the definitions of the alcoholic life. I was physically sick: my liver was enlarged, I vomited every morning, I passed blood in my urine. I was full of dread and fear, and I alienated virtually everyone around me. I was in the process of losing my job, and I couldn't for the life of me understand what had happened. I had tried, with varying degrees of success, to stop drinking on my own. At this point I knew that I could still stop drinking completely, but I was unable to control myself once I began drinking. The longest period of time I had been able to avoid a drink was five months. My wife was complaining about my drinking daily, and a vast gulf existed between us. She did not talk about it, but I knew that her departing the old homestead was imminent. I called AA, got the address of a meeting, and my wife and I went.

"How neat and tidy that all sounds. Within the first twenty-four hours of my stopping drinking, I had the sweats, hot and cold flashes, uncontrollable diarrhea, and a feeling of impending doom. I was so nervous that any sound made me jump. As I told my wife, my hair hurt and my teeth itched. But I went to a meeting. People were very kind. They shook my hand and I stayed for the entire hour. I was given a directory. When I left, I don't know whether I felt any better about not drinking, but I felt a good deal calmer.

"I attended AA meetings for four months that time, and I was cute as I could be. When asked to share, I would introduce myself as Ralph and say, 'Perhaps I'm an alcoholic. I'm an ersatz alcoholic. If I'm not an alcoholic, I act like one.' People were tolerant. Much to my surprise, I stayed sober for four months. I couldn't believe it. My wife couldn't believe it. No one at AA acted as if they believed it either. I didn't do any of the Steps. I didn't pay much attention to the ethical or moral implications of the program of Alcoholics Anonymous. I just went to meetings three or four times a week. One evening after being caught in the rain, I felt so good I had a drink.

"In the next nine months I lived all of the horror stories I had heard in my four months of sobriety. I couldn't believe how quickly things deteriorated for me. I was either getting drunk or going into withdrawal. My intake didn't increase, but I was less and less able to predict what the alcohol was going to do to me. During this period I traveled extensively, and I found myself going into withdrawal on planes and in inconvenient places in foreign countries where I didn't know the rules about getting drinks. My suitcases were full of booze and maybe a change of clothing. The fear and dread that I experienced during this period is difficult for me to describe. My wife acted as if things were okay, and I was into hiding my drinking on a full-time basis. She knew I was drinking, but it so frightened her that it was easier for her to deny my drinking than to confront me with it. We spent very little time together, and on the weekend she seemed to have a million errands, none of which included me. My physical symptoms returned in full bloom almost immediately and, in addition to my other maladies, I found that I could no longer remember events that had just occurred. I would read pages and not remember anything of what I had read. I could not remember anyone's name. I was going to hell in a handcart and knew it, and even more frightening was the fact that I simply couldn't stop.

"I called the man who had gotten me into AA in the first place, and I like to think my attitude was different. My approach certainly was. I asked him in a humble, breaking voice if I could come back to AA. He said that they had been saving a chair for me. I went to my first meeting that night. My bottom in this instance was not precipitated by any great event. I found myself driving to work one morning three-quarters drunk on two drinks, and I simply could not live that way anymore. I wasn't cute at the AA meetings I attended anymore. When I was asked to give my name, I introduced myself as Ralph and said that I was an alcoholic and desperately wanted whatever help could be afforded me. I have been sober ever since. I came out of fear and pain. Giving up was hard for me. I couldn't conceive of a day without drinking, and now I can't conceive of how I lived for so many years with so much pain."

Other bottoms come with less dramatic fanfare but no less pain. Becky B. described her bottom at a meeting geared to women. "My story is rather dull. I didn't drink very long. I had my first drink after I was married at twenty-two. I wasn't opposed to drinking; I just didn't have the time. There was no alcohol available in my state to people under twenty-one and there wasn't any around in my high school nor did anyone I associated with drink. My mother and father had an occasional cocktail, but that occurred so seldom I remember all of the occasions. Alcohol simply wasn't a big item for me to think about. I attended an all-women's college and was a serious student. I didn't know anyone who smoked dope or who drank, and so I did not smoke dope or drink.

"My husband and I dated through college, and he wasn't a drinker either. After we were married, my husband got a job through the county, and we settled down in a small apartment. I got pregnant; we had a child. My husband went to work, and I stayed home. I was never so bored in my life. I started attending club meetings and joining various civic organizations. I met women who were young and newly married, like me. Cocktails or alcohol punch was served at some of the meetings, and I found that I liked it. It calmed me down, and it didn't seem as if the baby made quite as much noise if I had a drink or two.

"I didn't buy my own alcohol for quite a while. The first time I bought a bottle, it was a big deal. It was a quart of vodka. I thought it would last forever. I went thorough it in three days. I began having drinks before dinner and some before lunch. Occasionally, I would suggest that my husband and I share a drink before dinner, but he wasn't particularly interested in it, and after a while I no longer invited him. When the quart was emptied, I bought a new one.

"This went on for two or three years until I noticed that I was drinking about a fifth a day and things were going to hell around me. The baby couldn't complain; she didn't speak. My husband complained that I ignored him. I didn't have much to do, but I couldn't get it done. I had started to drink to relax, and I was so relaxed that drinking was all I could do. I began having blackouts. Whole periods of the day would disappear, and I wouldn't know where I was or what I was doing. I was afraid of practically everything, and I never left the house except to buy booze. I was afraid to drive, as I was afraid of most things. I walked to the liquor store.

"Finally, my husband and I sat down and talked about what was happening in my life. He said he thought I was an alcoholic. I was shocked. Being defined as an alcoholic frightened me because I knew that I would have to stop drinking, and I didn't want to do that. My life had gone from being organized and manageable to completely out of hand, yet I felt I couldn't cope without alcohol. I had very little sense of what an alcoholic was, although I had heard the term. I knew that something was dramatically wrong with me. My family had no experience with alcoholism, nor did my husband or his family. He said that he couldn't continue living the way we were living and that our child was not going to be raised in that kind of environment. He demanded that I do something about my drinking. I told him that I would slow down or drink only on weekends. He said that he didn't want me to drink at all and thought I needed help.

"Within a couple days, I called AA and went to my first meeting. A lady was chairing, and she told her story. It was difficult for me to identify with some of the stories, but I had something in common with everyone I heard. I went to a seven-day detoxification program and learned something about alcoholism. When I was released, I began to attend AA meetings daily. That was quite some time ago, and I haven't had a drink since. My bottom wasn't particularly dramatic, but the desperation and the unmanageability that brought me here were as serious to me as the circumstances surrounding anyone's entrance into Alcoholics Anonymous."

The bottoms for these two were not particularly dramatic. Others have more dramatic circumstances accompanying their definition of bottom. I recall hearing the story of Nicholas B., whose creative driving resulted in his arrest early in the morning when the police came knocking on his door. He had been in a wedding the previous afternoon and had spent the previous evening celebrating the nuptials. He had a long history of drunkenness and had received two other DWI citations, which he had been able to handle with the help of a lawyer and the payment of some money. He had a reputation as a heavy drinker whose behavior was unpredictable. Recently, he had begun missing long periods of work, and he described himself as having difficulty remembering what he had done the night before.

During the arrest, the police explained that he had hit four parked cars in two separate locations the night before. He was easy enough to find because he had parked his car half on his front porch and half on his driveway. He had no recollection of any of these incidents. After sorting out all of the noise and thunder resulting from his wedding celebration, he found himself with two years of probation, no driver's license for a year, and a very heavy bill to pay. As a condition of his probation, he was required to attend five AA meetings a week. He did not come to AA to stop drinking; he came because the court demanded it. Fortunately for Nick, he was required to attend five times a week and have his slip signed and turned in to a probation officer. For this reason, he finally heard his story. He began to understand what had happened to him and what had made his life chaotic. It took a long time. He had never thought of himself as an alcoholic, but in the process of comparing his behavior to the behavior of others who were self-declared alcoholics, he recognized undeniable similarities. He complained that he had had enough trouble to last him a lifetime. He wanted his family back and wanted to lead a normal life. Nick has been a member of AA for the past five years and has not had a drink in that time.

The common thread in all of these stories and definitions of "bottoms" is that the individual has a combination of social and physical symptoms that can be explained only by alcoholism. Characteristically, the individual perceives himself as being out of control and is full of fears and dread. He perceives himself as having "lost his fit" in the sense that his past demands to be denied and his future is increasingly difficult to predict. The individual feels out of control. He may even think he is crazy, in the clinical sense of the word.

Rationalization and Denial

People who come to grips with their addiction to alcohol may have experienced many bottoms. As noted earlier, alcoholism is a threefold disease—physical, mental, and spiritual. The physical impact of the disease is ameliorated first (despite long-range residuals and damage). When people stop drinking, they feel better physically. Unfortunately for the alcoholic, his mental state and the quality of his spiritual life do not equip him to stay sober. In AA, newcomers are told such things as "Watch your mind. It's a snake, it will turn on you." "Don't listen to your mind—just do what you are told." "Be careful when you start to feel good; that's the time when you are most likely to drink." "Your body will start to tell you that it's okay to drink; be careful of that feeling." The early physical relief tells the alcoholic, "You're not that bad. All you have to do is slow down. You can quit when you want to." The alcoholic can rationalize virtually anything that will allow him to continue drinking. Remember, it's a disease of denial. For a person who persists in denying his alcoholism, the stage is set for the progression of his disease. The culture conspires in the denial process through a range of prescribed scenarios where drinking is encouraged. Friends and family all seem to agree that "You weren't that bad," "You're not an alcoholic," "You just drink too much," or, my favorite, "When your life straightens out, you won't need to drink so much." They too wish to avoid the stigma of a friend or family member who is alcoholic.

If an alcoholic wants to drink, any rationalization will do. Denial always serves to enable. It protects the correctness of the drinker's choosing alcohol in the face of varying contexts. Rationalizations are offered to families and employers alike. Let's list a few of these rationalizations or excuses and see if some sound familiar.

"We only had a couple of beers, honest."

"If you had my life, you'd drink too."

"Sometimes I relax so much I can't move."

"If I couldn't drink, I doubt that I could relax and be social."

"I drink only on the weekends."

"I can't have a drinking problem. I only drink beer."

"Sure I got a DWI; I was coming home from a wedding, everybody drinks at a wedding."

"That accident would have happened whether or not I was drinking."

"My boss drinks at lunch. Why shouldn't I?"

"I'm a salesman. I have to entertain customers."

"Crabs (or any other food) wouldn't taste the same without beer."

"I can't be alcoholic—I work, and I don't drink in the morning."

The list is endless.

Absence from home and avoidant behavior when criticized will bring forth tales of responsibility and labor. "I'm doing long hours for you and the kids." Meetings are replete with stories about picking fights with husbands or wives in order to leave the house in a rage and go off to drink. It seems alcoholics are frequently drinking *at* someone or *because* of someone. Drinking is never the problem. It is a by-product or a remedy. Rationalizations concerning work include reasons for not going to work as well as reasons for poor performance evaluations or for being fired. Such rationalizations are similar in form, if different in content, and they are meant to deny the consequences of drinking and to protect the drinker's pathway to alcohol. The self is never at the root of trouble. It is never alcohol abuse that is related to trouble. It is always something else. Anything can be defined as a reason to drink, and reasons for drinking all sound somewhat hollow. The alcoholic drinks to celebrate or to alleviate sadness. He drinks in the summer to cool off and drinks the same drink in the winter to warm up.

It is not that he likes what alcohol is doing to him; it is simply that it is the nature of addiction to deny. The addiction must be protected. His addiction tells him that everything else is responsible for what is going on in his life. It helps that he is not alone in his denial. Frequently, families are so resistant to having an alcoholic family member that they commit to any rationalization that promises a quick cure. To understand denial on the part of the alcoholic, focus on how the alcoholic thinks about his relationship to alcohol. One can hear alcoholics at AA meetings saying over and over again that they simply could not conceive of a day or even a short period of time in a day without drinking. If they didn't drink during work hours, they were sustained during the day by promising themselves a drink later. For nonalcoholics, this is difficult to fathom because they do not spend any time thinking about alcohol. It simply is not a part of the daily equation of their lives.

At a meeting, Billy B. told his story. "When I first came to AA and tried to get sober, I was advised by my new sponsor and others in the program to stay away from what they called slippery places, that is, places where I drank or places that I associated with alcohol. I found it impossible to stay away from slippery places because virtually everything in my life was associated with alcohol. I drank in the kitchen in the morning. I drank while I was in the shower. I drank on the john. I drank during the day when I was at work. I drank when I was reading. I drank when I was walking around the yard or doing yard work. I drank all night. I did not frequent bars very often. In fact, bars were probably the most neutral places I could think of. I couldn't even begin to think of a day without alcohol. I couldn't conceive of a day happening without alcohol happening along with it. It was as much a part of my life as brushing my teeth, combing my hair, putting my pants on in the morning.

"Because I was a maintenance drinker, I also knew the consequences of not carefully dosing myself with enough alcohol to keep off the symptoms of withdrawal. The cycle had to be interrupted, and with AA's help I did that. I lived with the withdrawal symptoms. I drank a lot of Pepsi Cola, ate a lot of chocolate bars, and did my best to keep my blood sugar level up. I shook and I sweated and I cried and I was afraid, but I didn't drink. I went to three meetings a day every day and stayed as close to people in AA as I could. They kept telling me that things would get better. The words were 'This will pass.' Finally, it did."

Sobriety is a collection of days, one after the other. For the alcoholic, it finally becomes conceivable that a day or even a life can go on with no alcohol. On the one hand, it is a matter of addiction; on the other, it is a matter of the reconstruction of habit, mental state, and worldview. Dramatic change in life experience is the result of both intention and action.

Frequently, the alcoholic's family precipitates the person's entry into AA. The family has invariably played a role in the alcoholism. Mothers and fathers have provided a home, food, and frequently spending money for a child incapacitated by alcohol. They deny or are unwilling to deal with the problem. Wives and even children call employers and creditors to make excuses for the drinker's inability to live up to his responsibilities. They listen to lies and remain silent. They witness bizarre, unpredictable behavior and hope that things will change. They need to know that as long as they stand between the alcoholic and the consequences of drinking, he will drink all the more. They are preventing the alcoholic from bottoming out. They are what AA defines as *enablers*. Some self-help books call them *codependents*.

When the spouse refuses to clean up the wreckage, vomit, and dirt that accompany a drunk or refuses to call the boss or the creditors to make excuses or beg for time, when the parents throw out the child and refuse to help him kill himself or to support him in his present condition, each begins the process of forcing the alcoholic to realize the nature of his problem and to do something about it. If he chooses to ignore the consequences and continues to drink, he will live with an increasing number of symptoms and social consequences that continue unabated.

Consequences force change. Alcohol is an unrelenting master. When the hat is passed at meetings and the secretary remarks that there are no dues or fees in AA, only voluntary contributions to meet expenses, people laugh. There may be no dues or fees for membership in Alcoholics Anonymous, but the members have all paid one hell of an initiation fee.

The Process of Getting Sober

Sobriety is a series of days lived a particular way. The alcoholic finally conceives of living with no alcohol, experienced one day at a time. In the cornucopia of solutions and alternatives, alcohol is no longer a viable choice. This realization is remarkable for somebody for whom there previously was no choice but alcohol. The process of how this change happens to the alcoholic and to his worldview (his fit in the world) is what this book is about. Although almost all of the changes that bring about sobriety are internal, the process of bringing about these changes is almost purely mechanical. Sobriety begins with acceptance. This means acceptance of alcoholism and all that is implied by that statement of condition; to be an alcoholic is to require treatment.

The Alcoholics Anonymous program is not for everyone who needs it. It is for those who want it. It requires going to any length to achieve sobriety. The struggle for sobriety allows for no reservations. For many, this is fine in theory, but somehow it never translates into commitment and action. To admit to being an alcoholic is to own the obligation of treatment. Such treatment often requires complete reorganization of one's life. The treatment of alcoholism is not the exclusive province of medicine or, for that matter, any other branch of the healing arts or social agency. In fact, the most successful treatment of the disease is nonprofessional. It draws its legitimacy from the successes of those who participate in its program and from those with long-standing sobriety who continue to attend meetings and serve as powers of example for those beginning the course of treatment and a new life.

Like other life-threatening diseases, alcoholism requires discipline to continue the abatement of symptoms. Alcoholism is progressive and continues regardless of sobriety. It may not seem reasonable that after a person stops drinking the body does not heal itself to the extent that it is again able to synthesize alcohol as it did previously. However, experience in AA indicates that alcoholism is a downward rather than a circular progression. Those who return to drinking after a period of sobriety begin at a point of less tolerance than they showed when they stopped drinking. Person after person who returns to drinking and then returns to AA describes the downward progression of returning to drinking as being far more rapid and devastating than the rate of decline before their first Alcoholics Anonymous experience. In every instance, they report that their lack of tolerance manifested itself almost immediately and that the compulsion to drink returned with the first drink. All report that after the first drink their drinking increased until, again, it was out of control. They repeated old patterns. They drank when they did not want to and rationalized it; they drank more than they intended to and rationalized it. Finally, they developed all of the physiological and social symptoms that brought them to Alcoholics Anonymous in the first place. Alcoholism is a disease of deception because in the absence of alcohol, there are no symptoms. Because the disease is so intrinsically involved with self-image and life definition, alcoholics are led to forget that they have the disease. If they forget the importance of their daily regimen and disciplines, they place themselves at great risk. If they drink, they will return to alcoholic drinking.

Earlier I discussed the literature of AA, cautioning that for the alcoholic who would recover, a period of reconstruction lies ahead. The framework in which that reconstruction takes place is daily meetings, and the daily regimen is the Twelve Steps of AA. It is impossible to work the Steps and stay the same person. It is impossible to practice these disciplines and get drunk. Sobriety, like alcoholism, is progressive. As time passes, it becomes as comfortable as an old shirt. It needs time.

Meetings: Why and How

When an alcoholic first comes to AA, he typically is full of resentment, symptoms, and fear. He is most frightened of giving up drinking. He knows what he will lose—what will remain? Belief is still lacking. How can anything as small as a drink be the author of so many ills and so much pain? It is a paradox to love and serve the very thing that is at the center of the pain. The imperative nature of the decision to seek help and to stop drinking is usually brought home at the first few meetings. With the decision, acceptance of a sort follows. This acceptance may be denied later or, more typically, reconsidered over and over. It suffices for the time. The decision to seek help is made when the alcoholic attends the first AA meeting of his own volition. He sees others around him with his problem who are sober and content in their sobriety. He hears their stories and sees how they contend with the various problems he contends with. If he is scrupulous about attending meetings, the seeds of belief and hope are sown.

The newcomer is told to attend ninety meetings in ninety days; he is told that sobriety depends on his total immersion in AA. I doubt that anything can quite match the look of incredulity and shock on the face of the average newcomer to Alcoholics Anonymous when he is told to attend ninety meetings in ninety days. Keep in mind that typically the person who arrives at his first meeting is in bad shape. He usually smells funny because no number of showers can stop the body from expelling alcohol from the pores. He is usually in the first stages of withdrawal or just a little drunk, scared to death, and, when told that he is going to have to rearrange his life to get sober, appalled.

A member recalls, "When I first got to AA, I sat in the back of a large room and listened to people addressing what I thought was a meeting chairman. I hadn't had a drink all day and I was feeling very nervous and was wondering what I was doing at this meeting. My former resolve had all but evaporated in the face of the kind of fear and psychic discomfort I was experiencing. When the meeting ended, I was approached by a tall, well-dressed man who held out his hand and shook mine. He introduced himself and asked me how I liked the meeting. It seemed okay to me, although I really didn't understand what everybody was talking about. He laughed and said that he hadn't understood it either when he first came to AA, but the important thing was that I was at a meeting. He wondered if I had a problem with alcohol and laughed when I said that I probably did. He said that he had never seen anyone in an AA meeting who was there by accident and that I would begin to feel better when I came to grips with what was happening to me. He told me about himself and his first meeting. Our stories were different, but somehow I felt close to him, and I began to tell him just a little bit about myself.

"Mainly, I asked him questions. I wondered how I could handle another withdrawal. Withdrawals had become more and more severe for me, and over the last several years I had avoided them by staying half drunk. He suggested that I keep my blood sugar up, drink Pepsi, and eat chocolate bars, but he said also, encouragingly, that this would pass and that everyone in the room had lived through a particular withdrawal and that things would get better. He said it with such assurance that I became annoyed. How did he know things were going to get better for me? God knows, they hadn't gotten any better in the last several years. That's what had brought me to this place. I began to wonder what I was doing there.

"Other people joined us, all shaking my hand and assuring me I was in the right place. My new friend invited me to join him at a meeting the following night. I felt pressured, but I accepted. I thought I could always get out of it later. I gave him my phone number, and he said he would pick me up. That began a series of meetings that introduced AA into my life on a regular basis. The more sober I got, the more I wondered whether or not I was an alcoholic. My body kept telling me what I needed was moderation, not abstinence. When I was told by people at meetings that it was necessary that I make a commitment to attend ninety meetings in ninety days and even entertain the notion of going into a rehabilitation center, I balked. I told them how busy I was and how my evenings had to be devoted to my family because I didn't see them during the day or early evenings, when I worked. I was told if I didn't start making AA at least as important as my drinking, I was not going to have a family or a job to worry about. As my alcoholism progressed, they told me to look at my record. Was I ever able to control alcohol? Was there ever a time when I took one drink without wanting more? The meetings constantly brought me back to my reasons for coming to AA. I began to identify with the stories I heard. I thought to myself that even if I'm not an alcoholic, it isn't going to hurt me to go to ninety meetings in ninety days. I ran out of excuses and just started to attend meetings.

"I expected my wife to complain about my going out every evening. To the contrary, she encouraged me. She didn't tell me about the agony or the anguish that I had caused her with my drinking. That was to come later. It was enough for the time being. She gave me all the support I needed. I now recognize, however, that even if I had not gotten the support from her that I did, I would have gone to the meetings anyway. I didn't get sober for her. I didn't get sober for my boss. I just got sober for myself."

Discussing the importance of meetings, Connie talked about her relationship with Mary, a woman whom she had been sponsoring for a long time. She said that Mary's quest for sobriety seemed hopeless. Every time she drank, she ended up in a hospital, yet she continued to experiment. She had difficulty admitting to herself that she was an alcoholic, much less admitting it to other people. Her lack of commitment to the program, according to Connie, manifested most obviously in her willingness to let everything and anything interfere with her attendance at meetings. Every time she found a new hobby or a new circle of friends, it became more important than regular attendance at meetings. She forgot that her sobriety was contingent on surrender to the program and doing things the AA way rather than her own way. She refused to see her willfulness as a symptom of her alcoholism. Every time she cut her meetings down from six a week to five, to four, to three, to one, she got drunk. Connie remarked that in the four and a half years that she had been working with Mary, Mary's longest period of sobriety was ten months. She said, "Mary always comes back to AA with full remorse and anxious to try again. She talks about her surrender as being complete, but almost immediately after alleviation of her physical symptoms, she starts doing things her way again. She cannot or will not relate the importance of meetings and Steps to sobriety. I don't think she will ever be a success until she does that." This pattern has been repeated over and over again. For the AA program to work, one must surrender to it and make it the centerpiece of one's life. As members say, "If you don't put AA first, you won't have to worry about anything being second or third."

The entire process of attending meetings and listening and rearranging priorities to meet AA expectation is purely mechanical. All that is expected or required is attendance at meetings. It is not expected that anything dramatic will happen, although at times it does. Attend ninety meetings in ninety days and stay away from a drink one day at a time is the mantra. The focus is not on "the future without a drink" or putting one's life in order or repairing family relationships. The immediate task at hand is staying away from a drink one day at a time. All things will flow from that.

It is frequently said in AA that the newcomer is the most important person at the meeting. He or she is ordinarily greeted at the door or inside before the meeting starts. People spot newcomers but do not overwhelm them. In fact, people seem to circulate around them. As an opener to conversation, newcomers are asked how they feel. Normally, they are not asked why they are at a meeting or anything personal. Instead, AA members will talk about their first meetings or about their need to get sober or about their symptoms. Generally, newcomers are told that symptoms will disappear and are given some sense of when that will happen. They learn how to keep the blood sugar up and not to worry about not sleeping. Newcomers are also given telephone numbers and told to feel free to call before they take that first drink. They will frequently be given a directory of meetings with some meetings circled where they can expect to recognize one or two faces from this meeting. They may be asked to meet someone at the next meeting. The important thing is that newcomers are made to feel that they are among people who understand and are willing to help. They are also repeatedly given the message that, no matter what happens, they must not take a drink. Nothing is so bad that a drink will not make it worse.

Although never stated explicitly, it is the consensus that change for the alcoholic begins with changes in pattern. This, of course, includes changes in the basic rhythm and habits of the drinking life. Everything awaits readiness. Change occurs when the alcoholic is ready. AA simply orchestrates that change. Change in this sense is all-inclusive. One does not think one's way into good living; one lives one's way into good thinking. In this chapter I talked about what actually goes on at meetings as well as the social and psychological implications of that content. There is no need to repeat it here, but meetings are the key to change and long-range sobriety.

The alcoholic is sailing in uncharted waters and does not know what to expect. Some are fortunate in being more outgoing and liking meetings immediately. Others do not like the meetings at all. They hang back and stay on the very edge of the meetings. They seem to resist sharing or discussing their problems. This reticence doesn't mean that they will fail at AA; it means only that their process in the program will be slow until they overcome their feelings and force themselves to interact. The program of Alcoholics Anonymous does not say that you have to like meetings; it says only that you have to attend them. That is the nature of the program. It does not tell you that getting sober is going to be easy or convenient or fun. It tells you only that if you follow the program, you will get sober. A careful working of the Steps and living by the ethical and moral mandates of AA will result in achievement of the Promises in the program. But for the time being, attending meetings will suffice.

5

MENDING

The Steps in Getting Well

This chapter focuses on mending and how the program of Alcoholics Anonymous works. The stories that follow are a composite of attitudes about AA and the recommended Steps in getting sober. They are presented in the form of a typical AA meeting. It is a sharing of experience and hope.

Joe begins: "When I was new to AA, I was in considerable pain, confused about what was going on with me and what was going to happen to me. I wondered whether or not any of the ideas racing around in my head would slow down enough for me to identify them. I wondered whether or not AA was going to work. I wondered whether or not my alcoholic career was ever going to come to an end.

"I liked going to meetings, but I didn't go to Step meetings. I was still on Step One when I said, 'I'm Joe, and I'm an alcoholic.' It wasn't that I had any reservations about being an alcoholic. It was that it implied what I had to do. Simply saying that I was an alcoholic wouldn't engineer a cure. Work had to be done. 'No more drinking,' I thought, but I didn't change. I went out and led exactly the life I'd led before but without the alcohol.

"When I came into the program of AA, I knew I was a drunk, but I also knew that that was all that was wrong with me. I was a good guy, and I had good qualities. The thing that kept screwing me up was alcohol. Everything else was fine. I had no need to change. The Steps did not seem to pertain to me. I wanted sobriety, but I'm not sure that I wanted to do anything about it. While I had no great commitment to one religious entity or another, I had no animosity toward religion. I didn't usually answer questions in terms of religion, however, or other unseen forces around me. That notwithstanding, I still hoped that somehow or another, my cure would be miraculous and I wouldn't have to do a thing about it. I would just sit passively and listen to other people tell their stories. For reasons I still do not understand, I decided to follow the form if not the spirit of the program.

"I got a sponsor right away and tried to cooperate with him. I had come to the point where I knew I couldn't stop drinking on my own. I was fresh out of answers. Recognition of my own ignorance was a beginning. I wasn't willing to divorce my intellectual orientation from the process, and if I got cured I was going to know the psychodynamics involved in the cure process. I was going to be able to talk about this. I was going to develop a formula for sobriety. I suppose I was going to be a combination scientist and sober savior. I asked my sponsor what I had to do. He told me that what I had to do was come to meetings every day and if I 'brought the body, the mind would follow.' He also said that it was not a good idea to think too much about what was going on. He implied that I wasn't going to understand very much about what was going on and that this wasn't an intellectual process anyway. I thought to myself, 'I understand everything, and I'm certainly going to understand this.' In any event, I got the idea early in the game that I could be somewhat passive about this whole thing. I thought at the end of three months I would be voted Mr. AA. I resolved to be humble. I resolved to let the membership discover my wonderful qualities. The important thing was that I had begun to believe in the possibility of my own sobriety. I had begun to put faith in something other than myself, and I decided I would go to meetings and listen to the stories. With some of the drunk-a-logues, I identified to the extent that I would say, 'I did that' or 'I didn't do that.'

"I took no joy in the recovery of others. I was far too focused on myself and my own recovery and its condition. The persons that I didn't identify with were the ones I was grateful for. They were the ones who were worse off than I was. They gave me someone to look down on or feel sorry for. This went on for a period of months, and it finally occurred to me that I had not had a drink for four months. Damn, how did that happen? I'm not sure that I had intended that when I came to AA, but it happened and I felt good about it.

"During this time of early recovery, I had been the most ornery son-of-a-bitch in creation. The wife was calling my sponsor and asking, 'Is there an end for this particular phase of recovery because if he keeps recovering this way, I'm going to kill him.' The truth of the matter was that my mind was just starting to wake up. I was experiencing emotions that weren't either dulled or structured by alcohol. I was recognizing the severity of my problem. I was waking up to the fact that I was engaged in a life-or-death struggle. I became aware of what I had done to my life and professional career, my family, and the people closest to me. I just couldn't handle what I was discovering and what I felt. There was no relief for the feeling. There was no release because I didn't have alcohol. Somehow it no longer seemed a viable alternative. I wasn't attracted to drugs. Something had gone on in the meetings. The stories and ideas that I had listened to over and over again had affected me. That happened despite the fact that I didn't think much about them and I didn't consciously try to identify with the messages. The platitudes, the quiet assertions of correctness that were in the literature, the simple statements of people that had been sick and now were well had an impact on me.

"The literature of AA said, 'If you want what we have and are willing to go to any length to achieve it, here are the steps we took.' I didn't think I wanted what people had at the meetings. I wanted change. I didn't know what other people had, but I knew that what I wanted was yesterday. What I wanted was my life back with all the material things, all of the prestige, and all of the social amenities that went with what I did for a living. As it turned out, I wasn't to have those things back, and it took about five years to learn the futility of trying to reconstruct yesterday and make a future of it. I've given that up but not without some considerable struggle. So the stories provided a number of things for me I didn't understand. I found myself changed. I found that I wanted sobriety. More important, I found myself increasingly willing to go to any lengths. That phrase finally began to mean something: 'If you want what we have and are willing to go to any length to achieve it, here are the steps we took.'"

Joe leans back in his chair and takes a sip of coffee. People are quiet. There is not the usual stirring around present at most meetings. Joe smiles and begins again. "Now you are stuck with it, aren't you? You've admitted publicly that you are an alcoholic. You've admitted that you can't do anything about it on you own. You have reviewed some of your own history, which clearly indicates that you can't handle problems with alcohol. After four or five months, those whom we have hurt the most see us getting better physically and begin to hope. They see us getting a little more psychologically unraveled, but they begin to see the possibility of change. They seem to develop a faith in the AA program shared by new members. In the beginning, I hoped it would work.

I was scared to death it wouldn't work and equally frightened that it would. The sober world was an unexplored territory to me. I didn't know what the sober life implied. I drank for twenty-five years. When people talked to me about sobriety, I wondered, 'What is that?' I didn't remember a day that wasn't associated with bourbon. What I saw in the eyes of people around me at four or five months was a willingness to accept the possibility of my change. I found myself surrounded by people who were wary of hope, people who were scared to death that forgiveness would be given, hope would replace anger, plans would be made, and then I would start drinking again and trash my life."

Joe continues, "It takes a long while for friends and families to trust an alcoholic again. That's why amends must be more than simply saying, 'I'm sorry.' That's why the literature of AA describes the alcoholic as a tornado roaring through the lives of everyone. It also says that it isn't enough to come up from out of the cellar after the tornado and say, 'Isn't it great that the wind stopped blowing.' A long period of reconstruction lies ahead. I think it is wise indeed that older heads in AA do not tell the person during the person's first year what he has to look forward to in terms of reconstruction. Instead the program focuses on growth and on the healing that is going on that day. 'Just one day at a time. Don't worry about what reconstruction is going to occur.' I knew in my heart of hearts that it was going to take one hell of a lot to repair things that I kicked apart. In fact, I doubted if they would ever fit back together again. It was a daunting kind of process.

"Here I was at six months with a whole lot of information I didn't want. I was helpless; I couldn't do anything about it. Booze was going to kill me sure as hell. People had read my future and clarified the direction of choice. I had seen other people go out to drink again. I was impressed with the fact that alcoholism is progressive. I could see it in my own history, and I knew that I was literally hanging on to a slender thread and that thread was Alcoholics Anonymous. I held on for dear life. What in the hell was I going to do? What was I going to build my life around? More importantly, I knew that soon the chickens were going to come to roost. All the crops that I had sown for the previous six or seven years were coming up and blooming, and I had to deal with them one way or another. I just couldn't say 'screw it' and walk away. That is the long and short of how I got involved with the Twelve Steps of AA. I did not willingly come to AA. I did not willingly begin to work the Steps and bring change into my life. I got dragged in. I was dragged in by my kidneys, my liver, my nerves, and by my shaking so bad I couldn't write a check. I came to AA because I had no other place to go."

A Secular View of the Steps

Joe continues. "Let's examine the Steps of sobriety in the program of Alcoholics Anonymous. The Steps constitute the ethnical and moral basis of the program, and to understand this is to understand AA. I brought an interesting complication to AA that hasn't gone away. I found myself to be a spiritual person with no commitments to a formal religion or a God. I had been a student of religion but not entranced by any one in particular. It was my feeling that I had made whatever peace I was going to make with myself and that others should do that for themselves. If their spiritual needs require gods, angels, mystery, Buddha, reincarnation, or a combination of these things, so be it. I would have to find my own way. The program addressed the question of God.

"Alcoholics Anonymous is riddled with controversy around the concept of higher power versus variously defined God figures. My first year in the program was spent in a constant fury about the people who got up and confessed their Christianity as being the cornerstone of their sobriety. I still get somewhat annoyed at that. I'm convinced that if the church or traditional religion had any answers for the alcoholic, there wouldn't be an Alcoholics Anonymous. The church has been around a couple of thousand years longer than AA and seems historically to have been concerned with more broadly defined issues. For a while I seemed to hit every meeting in the area that was full of revelations and miracles. I remember one meeting in particular when a fellow claimed that his 'higher power, which he chooses to call God' (I love that phrase) rewarded his sobriety with road service. His car broke down on the way to a meeting. Because of the intervention of this higher power, he broke down in the parking lot of a car parts store so that he could get the parts he needed and get to a meeting the next morning.

"The logic of this intervention seemed strained to me. Low standards often result in low performance—I personally would have expected a competent higher power to have prevented the breakdown or fix the car. Others in the program seem to need or perceive this direct intervention in their lives. Others appear to see a higher power as a source of strength or inspiration without heavenly intervention. We are many and varied in the program of AA, but all agree on the importance of a belief in something more powerful and important than ourselves. I don't get annoyed any longer at the confusion of religion with spirituality. With the people that I sponsor, the first thing I tell them is to get a conviction of a higher power, to get in contact with it and get comfortable with it because it is essential to the program. That power might be the program itself.

"Of the three phases of the disease of alcoholism—the physical, the mental, and the spiritual—I think that we repair ourselves just about in that order—physical, mental, and spiritual. The people I see who are successful in AA are the ones who have developed their spiritual life and spiritual commitments to a point where it is the glue that holds everything together for them. I see this spirituality reflected in their service in AA, in their willingness to help other alcoholics, and particularly in the performance of more menial service to AA, like making coffee, shopping, going to meetings, and so on. They serve the program by attending meetings that they do not need themselves or that are at inconvenient times. If there had not been thirty-five or so people at the meeting I went to for the first time, where would I have gone for help? I go to meetings just to be there, that to me is 'Twelve-Step work.' When that new, beaten alcoholic walks in the door, someone needs to be there to say, 'Hi, I'm Joe, and I'm an alcoholic.' Someone must be there to tell the newcomer, 'You can get better; it doesn't have to be this way.' There is hope for you; there is hope for all of us here in the room. That's why we're here, to share the hope and the strength that we get from AA.

"So, with this introduction, I'd like to discuss the Steps and what they mean to a person who doesn't equate religion with spirit, who doesn't use a particular form of God. How do you get around that? Given the wording of the Steps, I'm not altogether certain that I've gotten around anything. The discussion is hindered by a language that uses these terms synonymously. What I have had to do in terms of working with the Steps is to relate them to the concept of higher power and to those sections in the literature that discuss spirituality in neutral terms.

"AA grew from a number of philosophical roots, not the least of which was the Oxford movement. This organization was orthodox Christian in orientation and viewed sobriety, among other reforms, as coming through total surrender and confession of helplessness to God. Its approach also required a lot of praying and indications of devotion. Bill Wilson's personal history, including his gifts for mystery and revelation, reflect these roots. AA's cofounder, Robert Smith, had a far more conservative approach to the concept of spirituality. The result was a literature rich in both traditions. It is rich with the fabric of traditional religion for those who understand spirituality through this particular idiom. It is also, fortunately, rich in the tradition of spirituality derived from personal association or service, or from the individual's existential worldview. Sober, we deal with the how and why of everyday life. For us to stay away from alcohol, we have to turn our entire life around. Nothing in our lives can go unexamined. All of it has to be done on the basis of one axiom. That axiom is absolute honesty."

Joe continues, "Let us consider the Steps and how they apply to us in our lives.

"Step One: 'We admitted we were powerless over alcohol—that our lives had become unmanageable.' I had no difficulty with this Step. It wasn't happiness that dragged me into AA in the first place. When I came to AA, I asked myself if I wanted to drink every time I drank or did I just talk myself into the idea after the fact? I rationalized after I drank. I concluded that no one gets up at six o'clock in the morning and pours vodka in a glass, puts in a splash of grapefruit juice and says 'better living thought chemistry' as the sun comes up. People do not willingly do that. I did it every morning for years. One doesn't get half drunk before he goes to a dentist because he knows he's going to get gas and a whole bunch of other drugs. I wouldn't take drugs sober.

"Was my life unmanageable? Were things happening to me that I didn't expect or want? Did I end up in places where I didn't want to be? The answer to all of these questions was absolutely yes. Was I saying things to people I didn't mean? Did I deeply regret what I said and want to say I was sorry but couldn't? Yes. Was I hurting people who cared deeply about me? Yes. Was my life being eroded by a continual incursion of crises? My God, yes; when I was drinking every day, it was a source of excitement for me. What was the mailbox going to bring me? Phone calls? What did I do? Who did I do it to? What did I say? What did I buy? What did I sell? Goddamn, what was happening to me? It was excitement after excitement. I had all of the excitement I could stand. What I needed was peace. After being sober for a while, I remembered an old Chinese curse. 'May you be born in exciting times.' I had all the excitement that I wanted. My life was rightly unmanageable. No problem with Step One.

"When I came to Step Two—'Came to believe that a Power greater than ourselves could restore us to sanity'—I had trouble with the insanity part of the Step, but I had no difficulty with the concept of a higher power. I already had a higher power—alcohol. Alcohol was waking me up, putting me to sleep, and telling me what to do. Alcohol was kicking the soul out of me. I thought, 'Anything has got to be better than this.' I knew I couldn't stop drinking on my own. I had tried over and over again. I'd make two or three weeks and feel so damned good about it that I went out and got drunk. 'One won't hurt me.' Isn't that a nice phrase? 'One won't hurt me.' I've never had one drink in my life; I don't know if you've ever had one drink, but I never did. If I could have one drink before dinner, I wanted it in a pail. I couldn't understand why people measured drinks. Why have shot glasses? I measured it like this (holding his hand apart): how many inches do you want?

"I needed a higher power, I needed something; I couldn't do it on my own. I knew that quitting for a while wasn't any good at all. I kept hoping that if I quit, even for a few weeks, maybe my poor liver would say thank you and work a little longer. Maybe one or two of my kidneys would stop working as overachievers. I passed blood and other kinds of messy things. Boy, that's scary, standing there passing water in the morning and thinking, 'Christ, it's red.' How did that happen? Is there somebody else standing here? It's me. It scared me to death. I needed something—a higher power. AA was to become my higher power.

"Many of the conclusions I came to about myself were articulated after AA gave me a framework within which to understand my feelings. It was not reason but pain that brought me to AA. I have had more than one occasion to be grateful for not having to understand an action before taking it. I have learned to act on faith as well as reason. My belief in the efficacy of AA and commitment to its ethical foundations began as a need. I needed desperately to believe in something. I knew my disease by its symptoms and had virtually no measure of its depth. I knew its tenacity all too well. It's said that alcoholics seek an AA meeting when they have hit bottom. By implication, they are ready to ask for help. The incidents that precipitated my arrival at my first meeting are not relevant here. However, I did not arrive at that meeting full of humility."

Joe smiles, remembering: "I walked into a room full of people, delivered a lecture on how good booze had been to me, and told the people at the meeting that it sounded like a Tupperware gathering and asked where I could buy a bowl. I called them hypocrites. I railed on and on, telling them that they loved booze as much as I did and stopped only because they had to—just like me. Let's be honest. Let's talk about how much we are going to miss booze. We'll be miserable but sober and at least honest with ourselves and others. I said that my best friend Jack Daniels had died. I couldn't imagine a life without alcohol. I was sore at all of these people, and I didn't even know them. I finally just ran out of wind and sat down. I could only see sobriety as a black future.

"The people at the meeting talked about recovery and mental peace. They asked me to keep coming back. 'Will you meet me at a meeting tomorrow?' 'It was nice to hear you.' I went home and talked to my wife. I said, 'I cannot believe these people; you cannot insult them. No way to insult them.' I had the feeling that if I had puked in an ashtray, I would have been invited back. It wouldn't have mattered. They knew I was crazy, but I didn't recognize it. I felt something I could not identify. It was all but tangible, but I could not put a name to it. It took six months before I knew what it was. That emotion was hope, and I had not felt it for so long that it took a while to recognize it. When I did recognize it, it frightened me. I was afraid to hope that I found my answer.

"In spite of my bizarre behavior, I had trouble with the insanity aspect of the Step. How could you restore someone who was perfectly normal except that he drank too much? My sponsor pointed out to me that although I kept a full bar in the house and never hid my drinking, I hid the amount I drank. I was a sneak. I hid bottles all over the house. After I got sober, I found bottles in strange places. I found a quart of whisky in the spare tire. I found a quart of booze in my enlarger bellows—ingenious, absolutely ingenious. Who was I hiding the bottles from—what was I stocking up for? Insanity was drinking when I knew I was dying from it.

"My favorite story about my insanity occurred near the end of my drinking. At the time, my wife had a lot of annoying habits. For example, she used to come home at irregular times. You just couldn't predict her. That's annoying to an alcoholic. Sometimes she'd leave in the morning and then forget something and come back and catch me with a drink. I would have to pour it out and make a big pretense about drinking a cup of coffee. She was an annoying woman. She came home early one night. I had just gotten back from the liquor store, and I had half a gallon of vodka in my hand. (Never buy a small one when you can buy a big one.) She came in one door while I stood in the kitchen with the vodka, and I had an impulse to hide it. Why? Shame, guilt, fear of an argument, who knows?

"I jammed that bottle down in a fifty-pound bag of dog food. 'Hi, honey. Everything is going fine; nice to see you. You're home a little early, aren't you?' She walked right into the kitchen and picked up the dog's food bowls and chow scoop. That woman had not fed the dogs in years. I was stunned. I thought, 'What are you doing, woman?' She put the scoop down into the feedbag. 'Clank.' She knew that dog food doesn't sound like that. She put her hand in the bag and pulled out the half-gallon of vodka. 'What is this?' she asked. 'I don't know,' I said. 'Maybe it came with the dog food. You know, maybe it's an introductory offer.' She didn't say a word. She put the vodka back into the dog food and left the room. I ended up getting caught and lying like hell. I fed the dogs anyway. Remembering that incident, did I have any difficulty relating my behavior to the concept of insanity? Not at all.

"Step Three says, "Made a decision to turn our will and our lives over to the care of God *as we understood Him.*" My key was 'as we understood Him.' I had done a lousy job running major parts of my life. It wasn't that every decision I had made was wrong. In many ways I was successful and content with the roads I had chosen. I was, however, given to extremes in work as well as in play. I needed to be in control of myself and of practically everyone else. I felt as if I was swimming upstream all of the time. I never stopped to separate those things I could control from those things over which I had no control. I needed to control the reaction of others and all of the circumstances surrounding my encounters. It took a few years of sobriety to discover that the only thing I could control was me. I needed to flow with the stream.

"This Step required more than acceptance. It required action. Traditionalists seemed to have an advantage here. If you can think of an entity having a master plan for you, it is a simple act of faith to turn your will and life over to that plan or its author. If your views are less specific about authors and plans, turning things over is a more complicated business. The first thing I turned over to a higher power (in my case AA) was my drinking behavior. My will needed perspective. People around me needed room to breathe. I literally turned my will and my life over to the ethical and moral foundations and principles of Alcoholics Anonymous.

"I didn't know a thing about this kind of living, but I was to learn that I don't run things anymore. When I have a problem that I can't seem to solve or a decision to make, the first place I go is to the literature of AA. I discuss it with people in AA whose opinions I respect. I'm convinced that if I do what is ethically and morally correct, I may not get the immediate response or outcome that I want, but I will get the outcome that is best for me. I'm getting everything I need. God knows, I'm not getting everything I want. I'm still not driving a Ferrari, but it's not as important as it used to be. Maybe I'm getting better; I don't know."

A glass of water, a glance at his watch, and he continues. "Step Four says, 'Made a searching and fearless moral inventory of ourselves.' Not an easy task. I knew what fearless meant. It meant write it all down. But what was a moral inventory? It took a great deal of thinking before I finally talked to my sponsor about it. He said that this Step required that I identify the garbage in my life. I was to identify things that I was ashamed of, things that I wouldn't tell anybody about, and things that nobody knows about. Write it all down. I told him I thought he was crazy. 'I don't even think about that shit, let alone write it down.' 'Well, that's what has to be done,' he said. So I said, 'Well, hell, I'm not going to do it.' He knew I would get around to doing it and damned if I didn't. Because I felt itchy and peculiar about what was going on with me, I had to do something. I was not a volunteer for Step Four. I wanted to feel like the other people around me appeared to feel. I wanted to feel better about myself. The Step was more than a complex confession. It contained good and bad. It was a description of the themes in my life. It was the creation of a structure that made the patchwork of experience comprehensible. It provided a road map for change.

"When I got it all down, I felt better. The list was not complete, but it was as complete as I could make it at the time. With a great deal of trepidation, I considered the next Step.

"Step Five says, 'Admitted to God, to ourselves, and to another human being the exact nature of our wrongs.' In Step Four we identified the garbage in our lives. In Step Five we're getting rid of it and we're doing it publicly. We're talking about ourselves. In talking about ourselves, we can begin to relate to all of the stories and experiences we have heard at all of these meetings. We discover alcohol had led us all to similar places and experiences, to one degree or another. We lay the foundation for forgiving ourselves and in time letting others forgive us. We are at once unburdened and opened to change. We're not the best little boy on the block any more, but we're not the worst either. We're just one of the kids on the block. We no longer have secrets.

"The description of the exact nature of our wrongs provides us with the map of change in AA. But this doesn't mean it's going to be the only map we write. It gives us some guidance; some direction and impetus to move on to

Steps Six, Seven, and Eight. These Steps suggest to us that we be willing to change and be ready and willing to actively get in and about the business of that change. Step Eight says, 'Made a list of all persons we have harmed, and became willing to make amends to them all.' We're stuck with another list again. We must be willing to make amends to them only when amends will do no harm. That refers us back to Step Four doesn't it? Why are we making lists? Is it because we want to dig up all the old wounds and feel bad all over again? That's the favorite reason I hear from people who don't want to do the Steps. Why contact all of those people? They've already told me to screw off. We make amends not because other people are going to accept them; we do it to cleanse ourselves. The amends Step is for us, not for anyone else. The list gives a chronology of events and people. It provides a context within which to understand the behavior.

"Step Nine says, 'Made direct amends to such people wherever possible, except when to do so would injure them or others.' I've made a great big amends to someone whom I thought I had injured, and I was humble about it and wanted to apologize. Was there anything I could do to make up for it? I would be willing to do almost anything. The person involved asked, 'Who are you?' We learn a little bit about our ego. Maybe we haven't had all the impact that we thought we had. Maybe we're not as significant as we think we are. How did that happen? How did the most significant person in my memory ask, 'Who are you, and what are you doing here, and why are you saying these strange things to me? I don't remember any of this.'

"I've made some amends to people who have told me, 'I didn't like you then and I don't like you now. You were a drunken bastard when I knew you and now you're just a bastard, and it doesn't matter to me one way or the other. Get the hell out of here.' I thanked them for their kind attention and left. My thoughts were not always pure when I left, but I felt better. In making amends I had put some more unpleasantness and guilt behind me. We are not in the business of hurting people to make ourselves feel better. We don't make amends at the expense of other people. The literature of AA tells us that at this point in our program, certain things are going to happen to us."

Let's ask Joe to pause for a moment. His view of the Steps is centered on the "working Steps" part of the AA program. He is sober and intends to stay that way. His interpretation of the Steps is, however, influenced by his rejection of traditional religion. Over the years, Joe has developed a point of view on the Steps that is consistent with his earlier religious thinking and commitments. Some come into AA atheists and become deeply religious and progressively find themselves less committed to a specific religion and more to a diffuse sort of humanistic blend that incorporates a belief in a supreme being. Some remain agnostic. Whatever the persuasion, there is room for all under the AA umbrella of spirituality and concept of "higher power."

The Steps are defined as suggestions; interpretation and innovations are encouraged. For Joe, "higher power" is equated roughly with the group and the feeling of power derived from "people joined in working toward a common purpose." Differences in interpretation do not separate individuals in AA. To the contrary, these differences have served to teach Joe tolerance without condescension. He has learned that his way is not the only way. What is right for him may not be right for others. Lessons like these are carried over into the non–Alcoholics Anonymous world to become part of the new person in everyday interactions.

In his description of the Steps in his sobriety, Joe has described some Steps in greater detail than others. Given his secular bias, some Steps seem more applicable to him than others. We stopped him as he was about to discuss the section of the AA literature called "the Promises" and the last three Steps, frequently referred to as the maintenance Steps.

The Traditional Perspective on the Steps

A more mainstream perspective in Alcoholics Anonymous interprets the higher power in a traditional religious fashion. Keep in mind that AA was associated with a Christian missionary movement in its early years and that one of its founders was given to religious visions. Much of its early literature was couched in traditional religious terms. It emphasized prayer and posited the personal God, miracles, and a concept of a God that had time for and interest in individual problems. In its split from the Oxford movement, however, AA's split between dogmatic Christianity and spirituality began.

In the program's early codification, moderates prevailed in broadening the philosophical foundations of AA. The movement became spiritual and not religious. The stamp of Western European (even American Midwestern) Christianity can still be perceived, but it is tempered with tolerance and traditions that preclude particularizing the concept of "higher power." Nevertheless, at meetings one still hears, "This is a God-given program"; "sober by the grace of God"; "my higher power, whom I choose to call God"; and other expressions of religious commitment. People assert that God got them sober. Others at the same meetings will point out the inconsistencies in such a position and comment that if God indeed got them sober, then it was God who got them drunk.

At one meeting in particular, an older gentleman with some years of sobriety commented that he felt it necessary to defend the concept of spirituality from the encroachment of religiosity. He said that, from his own point of view, a God that gets a small percentage of alcoholics (whom he created) sober and decides arbitrarily to let the others suffer and die an alcoholic death, was capricious and not "a God nor higher power" that he wanted anything to do with. He continued with an educated discussion of the exclusionary effect of any specific religion manifesting itself in meetings. Fortunately for those committed to his perspective, nobody is excluded from AA on the basis of religious commitment or the lack thereof. He can be made to feel like an outsider though. There are majority and minority opinions in AA.

A person is a member of Alcoholics Anonymous if he says he is a member and wants to stop drinking. This means that people can continue drinking while trying to stop and still be members of Alcoholics Anonymous. Old hands in AA say, "Bring the body and the mind will follow." They also say with assurance that they have never seen anyone in an AA meeting who was there by accident. The wish to stop drinking is usually the underpinning for attendance, whether or not the individual recognizes it.

A Nonsecular View of the Steps

"One can never tell when AA is finally going to 'take.'" Frank D., in chairing a meeting celebrating his fifteenth year of sobriety, discussed his early years. He said that he had attended AA meetings at least twice a week for thirteen years before stopping drinking. "I knew that I was unhappy and that a major part of my life was unmanageable, but I couldn't get it through my head that all of the unmanageability and all of the pain was coming from that first drink or the occasional use of alcohol. Whenever I drank, I got into trouble. My physical dependency showed itself in violent withdrawal symptoms and frequent hospitalizations. I would come out of a drying-out spot and begin attending AA. I would keep going to meetings even after I talked myself into chipping, which is just taking a drink once in a while. Chipping for me inevitability led to a series of alcoholic debauches and daily maintenance drinking, which in turn led to more disaster, more crisis, and renewal of my AA-based, temporary sobriety.

"This went on for thirteen years. Then one day it ended, and here I sit. I've been sober for fifteen years. In my first year and a half of sobriety, I could not sleep. I couldn't lie down in a bed, but I would nap in chairs or lie on the floor. I shook much of the time and was unemployable. My AA information and support came from meetings. I couldn't concentrate long enough to read, and what I did try to read, I didn't remember. My short-term memory had been so profoundly affected that I couldn't remember names or connect them with faces or remember telephone numbers. When I wrote numbers down, I forgot what they meant.

"When I complained to people at meetings about my lack of sleep, I was told that no one ever died from lack of sleep. When I complained that I couldn't concentrate and couldn't remember names, I was told that the important thing was to remember where the meetings were on a daily basis. When I complained that I was unemployable, I was asked if I was sober that day. When I said yes, I was told that any day that I stayed away from a drink was a success and that things would get better. It seemed that, regardless of how I described my condition and what self-pity and pathos I brought to that description, the answer was the same: stay away from a drink and get to a meeting; things will be all right.

"It is now fifteen years later. When I am faced with the normal problems that everyone faces in a lifetime and I seek resolution or solace, the phrase 'Stay away from a drink and get to a meeting' rings in my mind. It is exactly what I do. I know that if I live my life according to the ethical and moral tenets of AA and try to be of service to other alcoholics and attend meetings regularly and lead my life to honest good purpose, things will be fundamentally okay with me. The Promises have come true in my life, and I am here at a meeting to share my strength and hope with you all."

Frank D. describes himself as having incorporated the Twelve Steps of Alcoholics Anonymous firmly into his life. He describes AA as the centerpiece of his life and maintains that if he did not have sobriety he would not have anything in his life. His sobriety comes before anything. Frank offers a more traditional interpretation of the Steps. In describing his program he does not equate higher power with God. Yet he makes it clear that he does not have difficulty with the use of the word God in the Steps or in the recommended , prayer aspects of the program. This description of his program contains no subtle criticisms of anyone's definition of higher power. When he talks about his program, it is clear what he is simply describing is what has kept him sober over a period of fifteen years. When Frank chairs a meeting, his quiet assurance and his calm are evident as he describes the chaos of his earlier life and his reclamation in AA. He gives the appearance of being a man at peace with himself. The Steps have indeed worked in Frank's life. Let us consider how the Steps are defined from this more middle-ground perspective.

Frank continues. "In Step One, 'We admitted we were powerless over alcohol—that our lives had become unmanageable.' In my experience, people who wonder whether or not they have a drinking problem usually have one. People without drinking problems seldom think about their drinking. It is not important enough to them to consider. The alcoholic can consider little else. Alcohol is always of importance to him. Alcoholics think differently about alcohol than nonalcoholics. These differences are not readily apparent in the culture because discussion of how we feel about the use of alcohol or drugs is not a part of normal, everyday social intercourse. How we feel about drugs is discussed more frequently than how we feel about drinking. For the alcoholic, drinking becomes equated with good times, success, feeling good, curing problems, providing the necessary social skills for normal pursuit of business, and so on. The more alcohol intrudes in his life, the more concerned with it he becomes and the more dependent he is on it.

"The First Step suggests that the alcoholic admit that he is powerless over alcohol. This self-examination forces the alcoholic to recognize his helplessness. The admission of that helplessness over alcohol is particularly frightening because it means that for sobriety to be achieved, alcohol must be forever eschewed. No one wants to admit that they are beaten. In *Twelve Steps and Twelve Traditions,* an official publication of AA's World Services (hereafter referred to as the *12 and 12*), it says 'No other kind of bankruptcy is like this one. Alcohol, now become the rapacious creditor, bleeds us of all self-sufficiency and all will to resist its demands. Once this stark fact is accepted, our bankruptcy as going human concerns is complete.'"[1]

Frank discusses this aspect of Step One in some detail. "I just could not get it in my head that I was powerless over alcohol. I maintained the belief that I could control myself and my alcohol intake for years. That single belief kept me drunk. Although I heard in AA that it was the first drink that got me drunk, I knew that I didn't get drunk until I had been drinking for some time. I honestly believed that I could take one or two drinks, or three or four drinks, and walk away and not have that amount of alcohol affect me in one way or another. I never stopped to think that this reasoning itself pinpointed how critically important alcohol was to me. I would go to any lengths to rationalize drinking, even a small amount. The compulsion to drink was so strong and yet so unrecognized, it was impossible for me to admit that I was powerless over alcohol. In many ways what I wanted from Alcoholics Anonymous was relative sobriety. I wanted to learn to drink like a gentleman. I wanted to be able to control alcohol. Now I know that the critical difference between me and nonalcoholics is that I have no control over alcohol and they do. When I realized that I was helpless and powerless over alcohol, I began to examine my life in terms of manageability. AA would help me manage.

"Although I still had a family and most of the trappings of middle-class success, I felt I was a failure. Moreover, I was about to lose my job. I was alienating people left and right and organizing my life around the availability of booze at different times of the day. My twenty-four-hour-a-day dependence on alcohol was necessary in order to maintain any semblance of normalcy. The difficulties and anxiety-ridden activities of day-to-day life were such that I felt that alcohol helped me get through them. I was to learn that alcohol was their progenitor rather than their solution. I had tried to stop drinking for periods of time without success. I found that if I woke in the morning and said I would not have a drink until one o'clock or two o'clock in the afternoon, by nine or ten in the morning I would be drinking, having rationalized the act. My ability to con myself was infallible. Attempts at controlling the amount I drank, or when I drank, proved useless. I was frightened and felt that I was on a downward slide that would never end. I was afraid all the time.

"When I looked at the First Step, I began to equate these feelings with being powerless over alcohol. My life was unmanageable and becoming more so with each passing day. At this point I didn't know how much trouble I was in. I knew, however, that I had enough trouble in my life. Later, I was to describe this as hitting my personal bottom. I didn't know anything about the disease concept of alcoholism, nor did I feel I had a biological vulnerability. It was no longer important whether or not my drinking was the product of weak will or moral weakness. I had to stop drinking, and I could not do it alone. I came to Alcoholics Anonymous."

Why do such discussions focus on the alcoholic hitting bottom before becoming involved with AA? The answer is that devastation is motivation. Bottoms are frequently beginnings. After Step One, the remaining eleven Steps demand the adoption of attitudes and actions that all but ensure sobriety. Who wishes to be rigorously honest and tolerant? Who wants to confess his faults to another and make restitution for harm done? Who cares anything about a higher power, let alone meditation or prayer? Who wants to sacrifice time and energy in trying to carry AA's message to the suffering alcoholic? None of these Steps appeal to the alcoholic who continues to drink. The motivation for Step work must be deep and strong.

After a coffee break and a stretch, typically taken in the middle of hour-and-a-half meetings, Frank resumes. He says that he is trying to speak to the newcomers in the room. He begins again: "Step Two: 'Came to believe that a Power greater than ourselves could restore us to sanity.' This Step is difficult but necessary for the alcoholic new to the program of AA. He has already admitted to the existence of a higher power in Step One. The higher power he has experience with is alcohol. If he is a traditionally religious person, this Step holds few fears or problems. He translates the power greater than himself into God and begins to relate prayer to sobriety. For those of less traditional religious persuasion, the higher power can be interpreted as AA, or the group for that matter, anything that the individual is comfortable with. The sticker in this Step seems to be the question of sanity versus insanity. Newcomers frequently ask, 'How can I be restored to sanity. I have never been insane.'"

Recall how Joe, at the beginning of this chapter, handles this question? He examined his own behavior and found that he did insane things. Insanity, for most in AA, comes to be defined as the individual's continually committing pernicious and extreme acts. Perhaps the most flagrant insanity is to continue drinking in the face of the violent symptoms that drinking induces. Insanity is doing the same thing over and over again in exactly the same way, expecting different results each time.

"Few indeed are the practicing alcoholics who have any idea how irrational they are, or seeing their irrationality, can bear to face it. Some will be willing to term themselves 'problem drinkers,' but cannot endure the suggestion that they are in fact mentally ill. They are abetted in this blindness by a world which does not understand the difference between sane drinking and alcoholism. 'Sanity' is defined as 'soundness of mind.' Yet no alcoholic, soberly analyzing his destructive behavior, whether the destruction fell on the dining-room furniture or his own moral fiber, can claim 'soundness of mind' for himself . . . Therefore, Step Two is the rallying point for all of us. Whether agnostic, atheist, or former believer, we can stand together on this Step."[2]

Frank continues. "Step Three: 'Made a decision to turn our will and our lives over to the care of God *as we understood Him.*' Perhaps the single word that unlocks the meaning of Step Three for the newcomer alcoholic is *willingness.* The literature of AA maintains that one has made a beginning on Step Three simply by joining AA and seeking help. By seeking help, the alcoholic is turning at least a part of his will over to the direction of others. He has discovered that alone he is unable to stop drinking. His plans have not worked out. It is time to turn some of that will and energy over to something or someone else for structuring."

The *12 and 12* suggests that neither the atheist nor the agnostic can legitimately avoid this Step on the basis of its inclusion of the word *God,* because it is tempered by the phrase "*as we understood Him.*" God or the higher power can be understood to be the group or the philosophy of AA or the program itself. The importance of this Step is that the alcoholic is willing to stop doing things his way and accept the direction of others. "Once we have placed the key of willingness in the lock and have the door ever so slightly open, we find that we can always open it some more. Though self-will may slam it shut again, as it frequently does, it will always respond the moment we again pick up the key of willingness."[3] In many ways, the admonition here is to stop swimming upstream.

Frank goes on: "It seems to me that, when we abandon our willfulness and go with the natural flow of events, a number of things begin to happen. We stop trying to run everything around us; we are better able to concentrate on running our own lives. When we stop trying to run the lives of others or attend to things that are none of our business, a great source of resentment seems to evaporate. As we become more comfortable with ourselves and others, people become more comfortable around us. We become predictable. The more we get our ego in perspective, the less it intrudes on those situations that have caused such difficulty in the past. The more we separate things within our control from things that are not, the more we are able to channel our energies into constructive effort. After a time, we begin to look at ourselves as the author of both our successes and our failures. This takes remedial action within our control, rather than a mystery."

AA members frequently use what they call the Serenity Prayer to remind them of the importance of Step Three: "'God grant me the serenity to accept the things I cannot change, courage to change the things I can, and wisdom to know the difference.'"[4] Frank's perspective is clear in his analysis of Step Four.

Frank continues. "Step Four: 'Made a searching and fearless moral inventory of ourselves.' What is suggested here is the development of a personal inventory in its most rational sense. Step Four is meant to encourage people to describe themselves as they are, without fear or shame. Some have referred to Step Four as identifying the garbage in life. In practice, Step Four develops into a kind of narrative of deeds, misdeeds, and feelings of resentment and frustration. The narrative is made up of descriptions of relationships both present and lost. In all instances, the narrative focuses on the actor's role in all of these events and analyzes his or her responsibility. This Step is the beginning of a chipping away of the armor that surrounds the behavior of the alcoholic. While the disease concept of alcoholism effectively placates feelings of moral responsibility for behavior, Step Four makes clear that while alcoholics are not morally evil people because they have been influenced by alcohol, they are socially responsible for what they have done. Additionally, if they are to remain sober, it is necessary that they change. Step Four is the place where that change begins."

Particularly apt is Frank's description of Step Four as providing a map for future change. The Fourth Step, carefully done, provides the alcoholic with a list of his most readily apparent character defects. He must learn to look for the cause of trouble within himself rather than in outside locations. If he is to correct the situation that has occurred or avoid unpleasant situations in the future, it's only his own conduct that he can govern. The assignment of responsibility or blame, in various degrees, in various situations, is inappropriate. He, as a member of AA, must take his own inventory and not the inventory of others. This follows because he is the origin of whatever difficulties exist in his life. "Therefore, thoroughness ought to be the watchword when taking inventory. In this connection, it is wise to write out our questions and answers. It will be an aid to clear thinking and honest appraisal. It will be the first *tangible* evidence of our complete willingness to move forward."[5]

Now to Step Five: "Admitted to God, to ourselves, and to another human being the exact nature of our wrongs." In all of the Steps of Alcoholics Anonymous, Step Five poses probably the greatest difficulty. It involves the sharing of deeply personal material with a comparative stranger. The sharing of such intimacies requires trust not only in the individual with whom we share but also in the program that demands the sharing. All of the Steps in AA are geared to ego deflation at one level or another, yet Step Five is probably the most crucial to the maintenance of long-term sobriety. "AA experience has taught us we cannot live alone with our pressing problems and the character defects which cause or aggravate them. If we have swept the searchlight of Step Four back and forth over our [drinking] careers, and it has revealed in stark relief those experiences we'd rather not remember, if we have come to know how wrong thinking and action have hurt us and others, then the need to quit living by ourselves with those tormenting ghosts of yesterday gets more urgent than ever. We have to talk to somebody about them."[6]

Confession in one form or another as a means of processing guilt is a part of formal religion and is found in the secular practice of various therapies. Sigmund Freud was particularly enamored of the concept of confession and the reliving of previous experiences emotionally and psychologically. He used the term *catharsis*. An intellectual reliving was of no therapeutic value without emotional content accompanying it. There would appear to be general agreement that we are better off talking about what is bothering us or what is going on in our lives. After talking about it, we seem to understand ourselves a little better. We feel a little less guilty and have a perspective on our responsibility in the various events that make up our lives.

The alcoholic does not approach the Fifth Step with another person, either inside or outside of the program, without a plan. The general content and the approach of the Fifth Step has been structured by the Fourth Step. Frequently, new material is brought into the process of the Fifth Step as memories excite other memories and bring more to the surface. Whatever comes out in discussion must be relevant, or it wouldn't have made itself important enough to be discussed.

The Fifth Step is ordinarily done either with someone who can be completely trusted or with someone whose confidence is already shared. I have even heard AA members talk about doing their Fifth Step with someone they are not likely to see again. One man spoke of doing a Fifth Step with a perfect stranger he met at an AA conference held near the ocean. They struck up a conversation, and before he knew what he was doing he was into the Fifth Step. The other person listened carefully, understanding what was going on. He has never seen the person since. Nonetheless, he is comfortable with his Fifth Step.

While the Fifth Step may be the most formidable to approach and the most difficult to do, it is the most immediate in its rewards. Over and over in meetings one hears testimonials to the impact of the Fifth Step. People talk about feeling relieved and of coming to the conclusion that they weren't as bad as they thought they were. Others realize that, as the Big Book suggests, there is a long period of reconstruction ahead. Regardless, all who have taken the Fifth Step have expressed confidence in their future as well as a sense of accomplishment. With the Fourth and Fifth Steps out of the way, they can proceed with the rest of the program. They have made a firm and positive commitment to their own sobriety. As the result of taking these Steps, they know themselves better and have a more realistic appraisal of the impact of alcohol on them and their worldview, and are perhaps, more tolerant of differences with others.

On to Step Six: "Were entirely ready to have God remove all these defects of character." This Step simply means recognizing the need to change and being willing to do so. In some ways, Step Six suggests yet another inventory. The willingness to change implies recognition of areas that need to be changed. This might be an appropriate time to consider the "double-edged sword" quality of most of our dominant personality characteristics. What is the difference between stubbornness and resolution? In AA the interactional context is stressed in making such decisions. In many ways, Step Six organizes the materials that were the focus of Steps Four and Five. Common sense is also a guideline. What would appear to be strength in some circumstances is frequently a hindrance in others. In many ways, Step Six bridges the gap between fear and courage. Step Six is a part of the reconstruction process. In its very simplicity, it impels movement.

Step Seven: "Humbly asked Him to remove our shortcomings." Because these Steps are close in intention and meaning I will consider them together. Step Six addresses the issue of willingness to change. The most obvious elements to change constitute a part of the Fourth and Fifth Steps and are referred to as character defects. Step Seven also contains an element of surrender. This Step is not an act of will but an act of submission and the inclusion of a higher power in the willingness to change. Those with traditional religious beliefs simply pray. Those with less traditional commitments can substitute the term *higher power* or *group* for the term *God* in the Step.

As explained earlier, these Steps are suggestions and not intended to hinder the process of developing a sober life. The key to understanding and working the Steps is willingness to change on terms other than your own. It is not expected that all defects of character will vanish or that perfection be attained. In this sense, it is the journey that is exciting and beneficial, not the destination. The AA literature suggests that for many alcoholics, the best that can be hoped for is slow growth and patience. The characteristic extremes, such as dishonesty, feelings of superiority and anger, the harboring of resentments, and even lust, procrastination, and selfishness, are dealt with. The goals we seek are old in the culture but frequently new to alcoholics. These goals attain a personal freshness in their inclusion in alcoholic's daily lives.

Teddy B., in describing his work with Steps Six and Seven, manages to include a description of change as well as what motivated him to change. "I was the West Coast chairman for the distribution of resentments. I couldn't see how harboring resentments against people who had done me ill would hurt me. I was not responsible for what they had done, but I was a damn fool if I didn't recognize that I wasn't wrong all of the time. There were a number of people who had cheated me and taken advantage of me in business and in my personal life. There were some people in my early sobriety who took advantage of my lack of judgment and my preoccupation with getting sober to cheat me. I knew that, if I worked the Steps, I was gong to have to apologize and make amends to people who I had harmed. I didn't see why people couldn't apologize to me and make reparation for the harm that they had done me.

"Steps Six and Seven mitigated against me. I used to talk about this at meetings and brag about the fact that like Dante I had created my own branch of hell for people who were my enemies. For each of these enemies I devised a particularly unique torture, and there were all of these little devils jumping around in this hell with pitchforks overseeing the various tortures I had created. At the meetings people just told me that resentments are dangerous, that they might well drive me to drink. They smiled and told me to keep coming back. You have no idea how annoying it is to be told that the answer to whatever problem you have is to keep coming back. I developed new resentments, and my particular section of hell got new residents.

"All the while I was carrying these resentments, I found myself getting angry every time I thought of each individual incident that led to the resentment. I couldn't help but judge people and in turn to judge the people who were trying to help me get over my resentments. It wasn't enough that I understood intellectually that these resentments were driving me crazy. I just couldn't see how I could let go of them. Fortunately, someone suggested how to let go of them. Another person told me to try to have good thoughts about the people that I resented most. I called this person a screwball to his face and told him to mind his own business. He laughed and said that was probably a good idea and then told me to keep coming back. I gave him a special place at the bottom of a molten-lead-filled pit, where he was to dip his tongue whenever he felt the urge to give advice.

"The more resentment I developed and carried around, the angrier I became and the more uncomfortable I was. There seemed no end to my dilemma, until finally I began trying to understand the people who had cheated me. I stopped thinking of them as something different from me and began to think of them as people with problems and character defects just like mine. I began practicing my own kind of discipline. Every time I thought about someone who had hurt me or stolen from me, I thought of someone I had stolen from or hurt. I was anticipating Step Eight, but I couldn't get off of Step Six until I dealt with this character defect. I had to find forgiveness for these people.

"My sponsor suggested that I stop trying to evaluate how much I was responsible for and how much another person was responsible for in a given set of circumstances. He suggested rather that I assume that whatever happened I was responsible for my own reaction and my own behavior and could not control the behavior of others. That provided the key. When I let go of trying to assign guilt to others and trying to control the behavior of others and looked to myself for ways to control my feelings and my behavior, I began to let go of resentment. This didn't happen overnight. This particular struggle went on for three years. I can say at this point in my sobriety that I have found genuine forgiveness for myself, and I work hard at finding genuine forgiveness for those around me. I am not saying that I still don't get my feelings hurt and that people don't cheat me and that I don't get resentments about it; I mean only that I don't keep them. My particular branch of hell is empty, and when my guests left, I left with them." Teddy quotes from the *12 and 12*, "'If we would gain any real advantage in the use of this Step [Six] on problems other than alcohol, we shall need to make a brand new venture into open-mindedness. We shall need to raise our eyes toward perfection, and be ready to walk in that direction. It will seldom matter how haltingly we walk. The only question will be "Are are we ready?"'"[7]

Teddy continues. "Step Seven is certainly easier for those who believe in God. The more philosophical among us relate this Step to seeking the group's help and relying on the ethical and moral foundations of AA. In either case, the end sought is the same. Steps Six and Seven intend for us to be better people and to live our life to good purpose. Step Seven focuses on humility. It tells the alcoholic that his values and his validity as a person lie within himself and not in the opinions of others or in possessions." Teddy reads again: "'Humility, as a word and as an ideal, has had a very bad time of it in our world. Not only is the idea misunderstood; the word itself is often intensely disliked. Many people haven't even a nodding acquaintance with humility as a way of life. Much of the everyday talk we hear, and a great deal of what we read, highlight man's pride in his own achievements.'"[8]

Teddy resumes. "It is difficult to think of any group of people who have made a poorer job of managing their own affairs than alcoholics. Independence and self-reliance are not what AA associates with sobriety. As alcoholics, we have lacked the perspective to see that character building in spiritual values has to come first and that material satisfactions are not the purpose of living. Quite characteristically, we have gone all out in confusing the ends with the means. Instead of regarding the satisfaction of our material desires as the means by which we can live and function, we have taken these satisfactions to be the final end and aim of life.

"The literature and the program of Alcoholics Anonymous make it clear that the same person will drink. A change in values and behavior is necessary for the attainment and the perpetuation of sobriety. Still goaded by sheer necessity, we reluctantly come to grips with those serious character flaws that make problem drinkers of us in the first place—flaws that are meant to be dealt with to prevent the retreat into alcohol once again. We want to be rid of some of these defects, but sometimes it seems to be an impossible job from which we recoil. Yet, we cling with a passionate persistence to others that are just as disturbing to our equilibrium."

As stated in the 12 and 12, "Then, in AA, we looked and listened. Everywhere we saw failure and misery transformed by humility into priceless assets. We heard story after story of how humility had brought strength out of weakness. In every case, pain had been the price of admission into a new life. But this admission price had purchased more than we expected. It brought a measure of humility, which we soon discovered to be a healer of pain. We began to fear pain less, and desire humility more than ever."[9]

Paul R., a university professor who has been sober eight years, discusses his involvement with Step Seven. He ruefully talks about humility as the key to his professional success as well as the key to understanding his inability to get along with other people. "Maybe it was because of my training or because of the position that I held as a professor and lecturer that made it difficult for people to disagree with me, but whatever the reason, I had opinions on everything. In addition, I had little patience with opinions that disagreed with my own. I found myself at odds with people and relished the conflict. I, of course, emerged victorious. I had a reputation for being sarcastic and having a biting wit. I thought this was an excellent reputation to have. I also had the reputation of doing my homework and being prepared to discuss virtually any subject at any time. What I did not have was sensitivity enough to recognize that people resented me, not for being right or wrong, but simply because of my arrogance. To be precise, the fact that I was right most of the time made me all the more detestable. I wanted to enjoy the company of other people and to share ideas. Others were not willing to take the battering this involved, and I began to find myself more and more alone.

"Because of my dependence on alcohol, this suited my purposes. By my definition, my isolation was the result of the ignorance of others and their unwillingness to see me as a leader and an intellect rather than the result of a personality flaw of my own and my inability to allow other people space. Believe me, changing a complete pattern of living and thinking is a hell of a job to do, but I knew that if I didn't do it, I would be drunk again. I tried to work the word *tolerance* into my vocabulary. After a while I tried to get the condescension out of tolerance. I began to listen to other people as discipline. I practiced keeping my mouth shut. It took all of the Steps, a good sponsor, and several years to get me to the point where I was willing to tolerate my differences with others and willing to allow others the dignity that I demanded from them.

"Old friends have told me I'm nicer to be around than I used to be. Some of them don't quite know why; others do. I no longer find myself defined as an argumentative pain in the ass, somebody to be avoided at all costs. My realistic appraisal of myself through the Fourth, Fifth, Sixth, and Seventh Steps has given me a fingerhold on humility. It began at AA meetings when I looked around and found others as devastated by alcohol as I was, sharing common goals and bonds and feelings. I began to think of myself as worthwhile outside of the external achievements and possessions that had previously allowed me to define myself as worthwhile."

Again from the *12 and 12*: "The Seventh Step is where we make the change in our attitude, which permits us, with humility as our guide, to move out from ourselves toward others and toward God. The whole emphasis of Step Seven is on humility. It is really saying to us that we now ought to be willing to try humility in seeking the removal of our other shortcomings just as we did when we admitted that we were powerless over alcohol, and came to believe that a Power greater than ourselves could restore us to sanity."[10]

On to Step Eight: "Made a list of all persons we had harmed, and became willing to make amends to them all." Step Eight brings to mind the sections of the Big Book that describe the alcoholic as a tornado whirling through the lives of others and, more particularly, the section of the book addressing recovery, which talks about a long period of reconstruction being ahead. Step Eight is the beginning of that reconstruction.

As Perry B. put it, "Looking back, opening old wounds, and carefully examining the history of pain that is the life of the alcoholic may seem pointless at first, but, like Step Five, the process is intended to cleanse rather than to generate additional guilt. As a matter of fact, to do Step Five and Eight and to feel guilt is an act of ego rather than humility. In evaluating the roles that others have played in our lives, the literature cautions us that we will be defensive and try to avoid examining hurts that we have inflicted on others. Right here we need to catch ourselves up sharply. We do not focus on what has been done to us. We do not define our behavior as reciprocal. We accept the responsibility for our behavior. Moreover, it is usually a fact that our behavior, when drinking, has aggravated the defects of others. We have repeatedly strained the patience of our best friends to the snapping point and have brought out the worst in those who didn't think much of us to begin with. In many instances, we are dealing with fellow sufferers, people whose woes we have increased."

Let us hear Roger R.'s description of his Eighth Step. "I was one of those people who maintained that the only one I had harmed was myself. Indeed, my family lived in a nice house; the children went to private schools. My wife had a checking account and credit cards and drove a nice car. I was at work most of the time, where I was supposed to be, and did a good job. In fact, I was promoted frequently. So I thought when I started making amends I should begin with myself. I was the one I had harmed the most. I mentioned this to my wife. She looked at me as if I had lost my mind.

"She asked what I thought she had been doing all the while I was drinking myself into oblivion. She described her fear and anxiety about my mental and physical health. She complained of the terror she went through every time I was late coming home or called from the office to break a dinner date and lie about an appointment. I had been so concerned with the problems of my own recovery and so involved with my own self-development that I had not taken the time to consider how my behavior had affected those who cared about me. My wife had never mentioned her feelings about my drinking other than to tell me that she didn't like it when I drank and that I drank too much. When she opened up about her pain and her anxiety over the years, I felt tremendous remorse. The literature had been right. It wasn't enough just to say that I was sorry. I had to do something about it.

"My amends began with my wife. Curiously enough, the amends began with my affording her the opportunity to vent her feelings without being afraid that she was hurting me or that the hurt would in turn lead me to drinking again. She talked about her feelings and the fact that although I had been sober for over a year, she didn't trust that sobriety. She was afraid to pin her hopes on my future. I had lied so often in the past, and I had promised so often that I would quit. She was ashamed of my being alcoholic and couldn't help it. She didn't want to tell our friends and was worried that her employer would find out about me. Rather than being offended or trying to register my own feelings, I examined hers.

"My wife's revelations to me served as a model for me to examine other relationships. I began a thorough list of persons who had suffered as the result of my alcoholism. I hadn't cheated anyone directly, but I had certainly been evasive and dishonest in many of my dealings. The list didn't grow to any great size, and none of the amends that I had to make were particularly large. The principal debt that I owed was to my family, and I felt that these amends were best made by giving them what they should have had all along, which was a stable, understanding person—one who could be relied on to live his life to a good purpose. I couldn't find some of the people that I wanted to apologize to. Everyone I spoke to assured me that everything was all right and that I wasn't such a bad fellow after all. Probably the most startling thing that I discovered was that my alcoholism had touched every member of my family, including my parents and brother. It had touched people only peripherally associated with me. In the process of seeking forgiveness from them all, I found forgiveness for myself in myself. When I completed the list for Step Eight and got started on Step Nine, I felt ready to continue my life in AA. I felt good again about myself."

Some, of course, will have more dramatic amends to make. The thrust of the amends, however, is not how they are received. Someone making amends cannot be guaranteed forgiveness, understanding, or, for that matter, even kind attention. The important thing for the alcoholic is the act of making the amends. There is the benefit. For some, the amends will be focused, at least initially, on financial reparation. The act of rebuilding one's credit and one's financial condition often seems enormous, almost unobtainable. Like all journeys, reparation begins with a plan, and it is the thrust of Step Eight to make that plan. In many ways Step Eight begins the process of ego deflation and humbling that is necessary for carrying out the amends in Step Nine. Step Eight can also be regarded as a mapping of fiscal and moral responsibilities. The Step also serves to remind alcoholics that they are not bad people trying to get good. They are sick people trying to get well.

Step Nine states: "Made direct amends to such people wherever possible, except when to do so would injure them or others." Step Nine is particularly important and tricky. It's tricky because its implementation ordinarily goes on over a long period of time. Alcoholics move around a good deal, seeking one geographic cure or another, and consequently people to whom they owe amends are frequently not in their immediate vicinity. Family members may have moved away. People may be hard to find. The Step begins with the list discussed in Step Eight. The list includes people of recent acquaintance and, if properly done, people encountered and harmed years before.

The point of Step Nine is not to run around the country digging up old dirt; instead, its focus is on getting rid of the garbage identified in Step Four, discussed in Step Five, and listed in Step Eight. The Ninth Step must be undertaken with great care, and it is necessary, as the Step admonishes, to be careful about not making amends where such amends would harm self or others. Caution and patience are the key words. It may be that illegal activities have cropped up in the life of an alcoholic working Step Nine. He must decide whether or not his amends is made official and involves facing up to legal penalties, or whether it remains unofficial, in the sense of repaying theft or returning property. Dishonesties and inequities in the life of the alcoholic do not disappear simply because he is sober, even for a long period of time. If he is to grow in sobriety and begin receiving some of the promises that are implicit and explicit in the program, he must divest himself of past wrongs and guilt. From the *12 and 12*: "After we have made the list of people we have harmed, have reflected carefully upon each instance, and have tried to possess ourselves of the right attitude in which to proceed, we will see that the making of direct amends divides those we should approach into several classes. There will be those who ought to be dealt with just as soon as we become reasonably confident that we can maintain our sobriety. There will be those to whom we can make only partial restitution, lest complete disclosures do them or others more harm than good. There will be other cases where action ought to be deferred, and still others in which by the very nature of the situation we shall never be able to make direct personal contact at all."[11]

Obviously, the key is common sense. It is important to keep in mind that the alcoholic must not make amends simply to feel better at the expense of others. The method of making the amends and the attitude surrounding them are as important as the amends themselves. In many cases, it is best to keep things to oneself, particularly when it concerns events that are long finished and whose disclosure would hurt people.

At a meeting, Bert F. discussed a man he had sponsored in the program. "I told Pete when he got to Step Nine to take it easy. He had a tendency to let his guilt run his mouth and was always doing the Fifth Step at meetings and in public. I didn't think this was the way disclosure should be handled and told him so. He was always so anxious to unburden himself, however, and had quite a bit to unburden. His wife was active in Al-Anon and had attended a number of AA meetings. She was supportive of Pete but clearly dependent on him and anxious that he succeed. Pete was able to do his Fifth Step privately with me. It was clear from the content of his Fifth Step that his behavior toward his wife had been abominable and that she had been greatly pained by what she knew. It was also clear that there was an enormous amount of material about which she had no inkling, and Pete said that he felt better being able to talk with me about it.

"During the Eighth and Ninth Steps, his guilt about his behavior toward his wife came up again. She figured prominently in his Eighth Step, and although I worked at it I couldn't get Pete to forgive himself for what he had done. I did tell him, however, that he would feel better about himself and the things that he had done in the fullness of time, that the Promises would come true in his life because they had in my own, and that he shouldn't be so impatient. For a while he seemed to get hold of himself.

"While he was in the midst of doing his Ninth Step, his wife began encouraging him to confess to her all of the things he had done. She cited her Al-Anon experience and her experience in AA meetings and said that she had already forgiven him for anything that he had done. She realized that much of what he had done was prompted by his alcoholism and his desperation, and she said that he would feel better and so would she if he confessed everything. He discussed this with me, and I reminded him of what we had decided. The things that his wife did not know about were history, and unless he intended to repeat them there was no point in sharing them with her. Despite her claims to want to know, she really didn't. Confession would only unburden Pete further at the expense of his wife.

"The next thing I heard about Pete was that he was dead. I got the rest of the story from his wife. With her encouragement, Pete finally confessed all. He told her about affairs with her sister and her best friend, about stealing from their account and from her parents, and embezzling from their business to the point of its bankruptcy. What money he had went to supporting a number of women and a couple of illegitimate children whose whereabouts he was uncertain of. I was familiar with his list of wrongs to his wife and it must have burdened her beyond her ability to bear it. After their talk, Pete had gone to sleep. She stayed up most of the night brooding. She got a pistol out of the desk that had been her father's, went into the bedroom, and shot Pete twice in the head. She turned the gun on herself but lived."

Pete's need to confess at the expense of others cost him his life and ruined that of his wife. Had he followed the spirit of AA, he would have understood that the expiation of guilt involves not only the forgiveness of others but also our forgiveness of ourselves. *It Works—How and Why: The Twelve Steps and Twelve Traditions of Narcotics Anonymous* is particularly clear about the objectives of the Ninth Step (which is the same in NA and AA): "The Ninth Step is not designed to clear our conscience at the expense of someone else. Our sponsor will help us find a way to make appropriate amends without causing additional harm."[12] The NA text also highlights the freedom to be gained: "As a result of working the Ninth Step, we are free to live in the present, able to enjoy each moment and experience gratitude for the gift of recovery. Memories of the past no longer hold us back, and new possibilities appear. We are free to go in directions we never considered before. We are free to dream and to pursue the fulfillment of our dreams. Our lives stretch out before us like a limitless horizon."[13]

The Ninth Step in both programs is the gateway to the maintenance steps—Ten, Eleven, and Twelve. It completes the preparations for the spiritual awakening that is so much a part of ongoing sobriety.

The Promises

The Promises comprise a passage from the Big Book which is often read at AA meetings. In the Promises, the alcoholic is told what to expect at the completion of the first nine Steps. It is significant that the Promises occur at the completion of the first nine Steps, because their presence in the life of the alcoholic is a measure of how well the first nine Steps have been done. In the beginning of sobriety, the Promises are read and anticipated. This faith in their appearance is based on the number of powers of example that the newcomer alcoholic sees at every meeting he attends.

In AA's Big Book, the Promises are set forth on pages 83–84:

If we are painstaking about this phase of our development, we will be amazed before we are half way through. We are going to know a new freedom and a new happiness. We will not regret the past nor wish to shut the door on it. We will comprehend the word serenity and we will know peace. No matter how far down the scale we have gone, we will see how our experience can benefit others. That feeling of uselessness and self-pity will disappear. We will lose interest in selfish things and gain interest in our fellows. Self-seeking will slip away. Our whole attitude and outlook upon life will change. Fear of people and of economic insecurity will leave us. We will intuitively know how to handle situations which used to baffle us. We will suddenly realize that God is doing for us what we could not do for ourselves.

Are these extravagant promises? We think not. They are being fulfilled among us—sometimes quickly, sometimes slowly. They will always materialize if we work for them.[14]

The Promises speak for themselves. They are not difficult to understand in content, but their emotional and psychological implications are enormous. Their location after Step Nine in the Big Book makes it clear that they come about as the result of hard work. The freedom and happiness promised are derived from working the Steps. The freedom specifically pertains to living free of compulsion and insecurity. We must keep in mind that alcohol shrinks the alcoholic's world and so fully circumscribes his associations that he literally is a slave to the psychological and physical impositions of it.

To be free of guilt is to be free of the past. The alcoholic is promised that his freedom from the past will not consist of denial but rather will include an understanding of it and its use in helping others. Additionally, changes in self-perception accompany the freedom from compulsion and guilt. As self-image changes, the alcoholic loses feelings of uselessness and self-pity as well as the selfishness that previously characterized him. A part of his recovery is helping other alcoholics achieve sobriety. As he gains interest in helping others his feelings of self-worth are enhanced. As he becomes more honest in his relationships with other people and honest with himself, he gradually loses his fears of other people. He loses his fear of economic insecurity because he realizes that he can control only himself and not factors outside of himself. As a result of this discipline he is content with his lot. His sense of validity as a person comes from within and not from external sources. For this reason, he is able to deal with life on its own terms. Perhaps one of the most important aspects of the Promises is the alcoholic's realization that sobriety is not an act of willpower but is in fact a collective commitment of millions of alcoholics following this program. Fulfillment of the Promises is the reward for diligence.

Steps Ten, Eleven, and Twelve are generally referred to as the maintenance Steps, possibly because they contain all of the elements of the first nine Steps and presuppose that the first nine have been done. Their emphasis is, however, on a daily progression. The additional element in these three Steps is an emphasis on spirituality. "We have entered the world of the Spirit. Our next function is to grow in understanding and effectiveness. This is not an overnight matter. It should continue for our lifetime."[15]

Significantly, the literature goes on to say that the beginning of Step Ten assumes that the alcoholic has stopped fighting or resisting anything, including alcohol. He is no longer concerned with the struggle to avoid drinking so much as he is concerned with the construction of a life that precludes drinking as a possibility. In this regard, the literature says that, "if tempted, we recoil from it as from a hot flame."[16]

Step Ten: "Continued to take personal inventory and when we were wrong promptly admitted it." The daily inventory of the alcoholic is not constant fault-finding with self or with one's actions. Instead, this inventory is a way to establish an internal barometer of emotional and spiritual well-being. Nonalcoholics develop these senses as part of their every day socialization. Because alcohol strongly impairs the normal learning process, the alcoholic does not learn to be sensitive to his daily experiences. In this Step, as in the working of all of the Steps, the purpose is to maintain an even keel and a lifestyle that nourishes sobriety. It is important for alcoholics to be aware that they are at risk. "A continuous look at our assets and liabilities, and a real desire to learn and grow by this means, are necessities for us. We alcoholics have learned this the hard way. More experienced people, of course, in all times and places have practiced unsparing self-survey and criticism. For the wise have always known that no one can make much of his life until self-searching becomes a regular habit, until he is able to admit and accept what he finds, and until he patiently and persistently tries to correct what is wrong . . . [E]motional hangover [is] the direct result of yesterday's and sometimes today's excesses of negative emotion—anger, fear, jealousy, and the like. If we would live serenely today and tomorrow, we certainly need to eliminate these hangovers."[17]

Joe was just about to discuss Step Ten. "When I got to the end of Step Nine, I felt a lot better. Some of the Promises were coming true in my life. I felt better about myself, and I understood my past. I had begun working with newcomers in the program and found myself of all people sponsoring others in the program. Although I wasn't certain that I had done an adequate Fourth Step, I was so caught up in the daily activities of living my life and going to meetings that I wasn't thinking much about myself. I had Step Ten in my daily life without thinking much about it. I began my day by being grateful when I awoke that I had been safe and sober the day before. I renewed my conviction every morning that I was going to be sober for this day. Since I had been sober, it had been my habit to keep a list of things that I had to do during the day. Additionally, I read over my list and planned what AA meeting I was going to attend. The meetings that I attended during the week depended on who I was sponsoring and where my network of friends would be. At times I varied meetings just for the sake of variety.

"I used the ease with which I was able to interact with others as a measure of the quality of my program in Alcoholics Anonymous. This pertains to one of the most annoying axioms I found in the AA program when I was first getting sober. As I said earlier, getting sober is healthy and in the long run good for you, but no one promises that it is going to be convenient. I found this spiritual axiom to be the most inconvenient of all. Stated simply—if you have trouble with someone or something, the trouble lies within you. It meant that every time I had a blowup of one kind or another, I had to take a look at myself. I couldn't blame other people for how I felt or for what happened to me. It reinforced those parts of the program that addressed my egocentricity and my attempts at controlling everyone and everything around me. With this axiom in mind, the only thing I could change was myself.

"This put a lot of responsibility on me. For some reason or another it always seemed easier for me to rearrange the world to suit my moods and needs rather then to change my moods or my needs. Sobriety has helped me reorganize that particular set of priorities, and the spiritual axiom has become a part of my daily inventory. I have come to believe that self-righteous anger and resentment are two things that the alcoholic simply cannot tolerate in his daily life. I think both of them lead to drinking. When I find myself getting angry about a situation, I do my best to leave it. When I can't leave a particularly provocative situation, I close my eyes and meditate for a little while and try to isolate myself from my emotions. Believe it or not, it works. As far as resentments are concerned, I do my best to have good thoughts about people that I begin to feel resentment toward.

"My resentments have never affected anyone except myself. The result of my thinking good things about the people who have hurt me is that I will feel better. This is true of other emotions such as jealousy, envy, self-pity, hurt, pride, and so on. The literature describing Step Ten suggested that it was necessary for me to develop self-restraint. At first, this was difficult. It was my habit to try to take care of things immediately, which usually meant that I jumped right into the middle of things that I couldn't control and so muddied the waters that it was impossible to resolve any situation. I, of course, ended up double frustrated in such situations. This is what I meant when I said I spent most of my life swimming upstream. I was always out of step and going the wrong way, and it seemed to me the best way to take care of that now was to march with people rather than against them. I don't write letters I regret anymore. I don't say things out of anger I deeply regret anymore. I don't make nasty phone calls. I try not to be critical, and I try to find good things to note about people. As a matter of fact, today, when I look at what other people do, I automatically assume that they are doing the best they can. When you see people in that light, it's hard to resent them for what they are not doing.

"I've had a lot of pain and difficulty in my life since I got sober. A lot of my chickens came home to roost. I lost the right to participate in my profession and have had to adjust to that. I don't know if that will ever change. This has been a source of pain and yet a source of enforced growth in my life. I have had to separate the things I could control from the things over which I have no control. At this point in my sobriety, I am convinced that if I continue to lead my life to good purpose, things will be basically all right with me. I guess what I am saying is that things will be the way they ought to be.

"One of the most important parts of Step Ten was admitting when I was wrong. I began with my wife. I did it just because it annoyed the hell out of her. She was not accustomed to having me admit that I was wrong. To the contrary, she was accustomed to me analyzing situations and carefully parceling out responsibility and appropriate portions of guilt. When I stopped doing that and began admitting I was wrong, she was shocked. She would immediately forgive me and wouldn't bring up the subject matter again. She just didn't know how to deal with it. I don't think she liked it. After a while, it was becoming clear that this was a way of life. I stopped taking delight in her consternation and began following the immediate admission of responsibility with changes in behavior. I noticed that I wasn't making the same mistakes over and over again. Evidently, I was still capable of learning. I have found also that most mature people who have made their compromises and adjustments with life's processes do exactly the same thing. They do not live in a world that is defined in black and white. They accept responsibility for their own behavior, and they do not expect that they will be correct 100 percent of the time. Their ego is not on the line every time they admit they are wrong. To the contrary, it is an expected part of their day."

According to the 12 and 12, "Finally, we begin to see that all people, including ourselves, are to some extent emotionally ill as well as frequently wrong, and then we approach true tolerance and see what real love for our fellows actually means. It will become more and more evident as we go forward that it is pointless to become angry, or to get hurt by people who, like us, are suffering from the pains of growing up."[18]

Step Eleven: "Sought through prayer and meditation to improve our conscious contact with God *as we understood Him,* praying only for knowledge of His will for us and the power to carry that out." Like all the other Steps, the intent of Step Eleven is quite clear. Prayer and meditation are suggested to cover those with religious commitments and those without specific religious commitments. Both meditation and prayer suggest a time set aside in the day for inner and outer calm. Meditation and prayer are not to be confused with inventory taking. This is the time for nurturing a sense of spirituality and comfort with manifest growth. I have heard a number of people at meetings say that their meditation time is largely spent in gratitude. These people seem to feel that gratitude constitutes a wellspring of strength and a buffer between the normal vicissitudes of daily life and the self.

It is difficult to describe how this Step manifests itself in the life of the alcoholic. It has been described variously as magic or damned mysterious. After a period of sobriety and a period of meditation, solutions sought to life's problems are guided by the moral and spiritual principles of AA. Our solutions are selfless and other-directed. Life in this context seems to become rich and full and less confusing. I think it is fair to say that as life becomes richer, it becomes simpler. As a friend said, "There just don't seem to be that many decisions to make."

Step Twelve: "Having had a spiritual awakening as the result of these steps, we tried to carry this message to alcoholics, and to practice these principles in all our affairs." As the literature says, Step Twelve is about the joy of living. On the one hand it speaks of the spiritual awakening and by implication the spiritual life of the alcoholic who has effectively worked the first eleven Steps. The alcoholic carries a message to alcoholics who still suffer (that is, still drink), by virtue of being a "power of example" in sobriety. It is often asked, how can the program remain anonymous and at the same time be a program based on attraction? The answer is obvious; alcoholics in AA are anonymous in varying degrees. Some are anonymous to all but their closest friends. Others are anonymous to the world outside of AA. Some are anonymous to virtually no one. Others speak openly about their addiction and life in AA but are careful to maintain their anonymity.

Ethan L. offered the following: "In my own case I couldn't remain particularly anonymous. I found AA because of an ad on television. I wondered how many would be as fortunate as I was. When I got sober I told all of my friends about my life in AA. I did this for two reasons. To begin with, I wanted them to know that there would be changes in me and that I wouldn't be drinking around them. Second of all, I wanted the protection of having them know that I was an alcoholic so that if I ever did ask them for a drink or try to drink around them, they would ask me what in the hell was the matter with me and what was I doing. I needed all the help and all the protection I could get. So a lot of people knew about me from my first involvement in AA. I found that it worked, and in related social activities, most particularly church activities, my identification as a recovered alcoholic allowed people to talk with me about their own drinking problems or the drinking problems of other family members. My experience and life have brought a good number of people into AA and some have stayed sober." What is significant is leading a life to good purpose.

Joe picks up the narrative: "Having moral and ethical principles in one's life is not the product of an intellectual exercise. One does not think one's way into good living. One lives one's way into good thinking. The recovering alcoholic must live his life on the basis of honesty. He must be honest in his evaluation of himself. He must offer himself in service to other alcoholics who still suffer and must keep in mind that this service is selflessly given and acts to maintain his own sobriety.

"The longer I am in AA the more I realize the importance of sharing my sobriety and my way of life with other people. My sense of serenity and well-being comes from practicing the Twelve Steps absolutely and following without question the moral and ethical precepts that are embodied in them. I don't question whether or not I should be charitable and kind toward other people. I like to think that I do it automatically now. This doesn't mean that I don't have hassles and ups and downs, because I do. It just means that they mean different things to me and that I handle them differently. Before I came to AA, I was drunk all the time. Since coming to AA, I haven't been drunk. There has to be a connection.

"I am grateful on a day-to-day basis for the benefits of the new life and the emotional and spiritual comfort that I find therein. I find myself talking unashamedly about topics such as morals and kindness and love and sharing what previously would have embarrassed me. I frequently find myself amazed at the changes in my attitudes. I work hard at AA. I go to six to seven meetings a week and try to help other alcoholics. I am secretary at meetings where I can be; I share when I am called on. I make coffee and put away chairs. I am part of the solutions in my life. After all, our problems were of our own making. Besides, we have stopped fighting anybody or anything. We have to."

6

THE COMPONENTS OF SOBRIETY

One of the principal components in attaining and sustaining sobriety is regular attendance at meetings. Other components include obtaining a sponsor and reading all of the AA literature, particularly *Alcoholics Anonymous* (the Big Book). A sponsor is an important element of anyone's ongoing program. It is particularly important during the first year of sobriety, when first attempts are being made at Steps One through Five. People do Steps at their own speed and depending on the sponsor's sense of timing. The first year of sobriety may include focus on any number of Steps. As it is said in the program, "We are many and varied." In any case, a sponsor facilitates the process.

Sponsorship

There is a formal way of getting a sponsor in AA. It is formal for a reason. Newcomers to AA will frequently use as sponsors people that they have met at meetings without formalizing the relationship. This can work for a while, but it is important that the newcomer formally ask someone to be a sponsor. The process of asking is an essential part of the sponsorship configuration. By asking someone to be a sponsor, the individual simultaneously admits his dependence on things outside of himself for sobriety, shows his willingness to be cooperative, and acknowledges that someone may know more about getting sober than he does. The Steps in AA involve acceptance, some degree of humility, and a willingness to take direction. Frequently, it is at this point that AA's program of ego deflation begins. To ask someone to be your sponsor in AA is to invite him into your life. Sponsors are given certain privileges of communication and inquiry. Their questions are to be answered, and their directions and suggestions are to be followed. It is good for the newcomer to remember that his sponsor also has a sponsor in AA. In addition to giving suggestions, sponsors are friends and confidants, available for good listening or advice on virtually all matters. Sponsors are decidedly partisan. They are on the side of the sobriety of the people they sponsor.

Paula reports, "I was in the program for about four months. I had been talking to one of the first people I had met in AA about my progress in the program. I talked about my anxieties, fears, and concerns about sobriety and what was happening to me in general. I was comfortable in the arrangement, but I had been around long enough to know that the basic AA program included having a sponsor. I felt that I had one.

"One evening at a meeting, I began my usual discussion of what was going on with me. The lady stopped me and asked if it would be more proper for me to discuss these things with a sponsor. I said, 'I thought you were my sponsor.' She said, 'You haven't asked me.' I was taken aback. Her attitude wasn't hostile so much as it was instructive. I said that I had assumed that she was my sponsor. She seemed to have been acting like a sponsor, and I had certainly used her like one. She explained that that wasn't the way the program worked. I asked her if she would be my sponsor. I thought that would put an end to it. She said she wanted to think about it for a day or two.

"I was hurt. I felt that she should have said yes immediately, but I didn't say anything. I waited for three days before I asked her what she'd decided. She said she would act as my sponsor officially for a year, at which time we would have to reassess the effectiveness of our relationship. She gave my hand a little squeeze. I really felt better.

"Somehow or the other the relationship changed. I wasn't just talking to a friend at a meeting. I was talking to my sponsor. The nature of our conversations didn't change in content but in terms of impact. I found myself resisting advice, arguing about things, doing a number of things I would have not done with someone that I did not have a formal arrangement with. I discovered that I had invited this person into my life in a very special kind of way. It was only much later in the development of my program that I realized how important the formal process of asking a sponsor to act in that role was.

"I asked people at meetings where sponsors got all this wisdom. It seemed to me that because anyone in AA could act as anyone else's sponsor, it implied that a lot of ordinary people would be offering advice on a variety of subjects that they were not qualified to address. What I had missed in my assessment of the role of sponsorship was that the sponsor was ordinarily a person with a few years of sobriety. They advise on subjects they are knowledgeable about with regard to alcoholism and the program. In a way, they reflect the collected wisdom of the group."

Newcomers are advised to pick their sponsors carefully, to find someone with whom they feel affinity, for whom they have some respect, and whose sobriety they admire. They are cautioned also to try to find people with whom they are compatible. More importantly, they are told to "stick with the winners," that is, to find those people whose behavior and continuous attendance at meetings reflect the impact of the program of Alcoholics Anonymous in their lives. Familiarity with the program and continuous attendance at AA meetings will make such persons readily discernible. While length of sobriety is important, it is not the sole criteria. If length of sobriety is mentioned at all by numbers of years, it is mentioned in passing.

Individuals are, however, encouraged to celebrate anniversaries at the completion of each year of sobriety. These are called "power of example" meetings. The person celebrating the anniversary chairs the meeting and afterwards is presented with a token, usually a metal disk with the number of years sober engraved on it, and a large anniversary cake. Anniversary meetings have a definite party atmosphere to them. Members of AA take particular joy in the sobriety of fellow members. Power of example meetings demonstrate to newcomers that long sobriety is possible. For those experienced in the program, anniversary meetings reaffirm their own commitment.

Beyond the number of years of sobriety, the quality of sobriety or the depth of spirituality or commitment are important criteria in the choice of a sponsor. "Some people just seem to glow with it." AA sponsors draw wisdom from the experiences, strength, and solutions they have heard discussed at other meetings by other alcoholics with similar problems. This is the basis of their advice.

All solutions and approaches to problems are outlined, in the most general sense of that word, in the AA literature. The Twelve Steps and the Twelve Traditions offer general guides to behavior, and it is usually only the specifics of a situation that need to be sorted out. Sponsors are as committed to the Steps and the moral and ethical traditions of AA as are the people they sponsor. If they do not know a solution to a given situation, they will share that and try to help find a source for additional information or seek additional consultation.

Sponsors are not gods, and they are not expected to act godlike. Their role is to mentor and support.

People frequently have the solution to their problems but resist that solution because it is inconvenient or because they want reassurance about what they are going to do. Their concern is often not the immediate solution so much as the relationship of that solution to sobriety. For people who are serious about getting sober, sobriety is the centerpiece of their lives. Maintaining sobriety precedes the consideration of any solution to a given problem. Solutions are weighed against their impact on sobriety. When people say that AA is an honest program, they are saying that honesty is the foundation on which all sobriety is based. Any solution to a problem which compromises honesty, be it a business problem or a personal problem, will therefore compromise sobriety. Dishonesty places the alcoholic at risk.

Bill B. recalls, "I had been in AA three or four months when I tried to get a sponsor. I asked a man who I had heard chair several meetings. He looked square as hell but seemed to have a pretty good sense of who he was and what he was doing. He had been sober for about three years. He was a machinist by profession, and I thought that his approach would be more basic and perhaps less complicated than someone with more education. I knew I was superior to him in that department, and I assumed I was in a lot of others. But I asked anyway.

"He said he wanted to think about it. I got pissed, but he thought about it anyway. About a week later, he said that he would be glad to be my sponsor and handed me a list of things he wanted me to read. I took the list but with a lot of reservations. I wondered why in the hell I had picked this guy. As it turned out, he was just right for me. I read what he suggested and discussed it with him. I found that his understanding of sobriety was far greater than mine, and I discovered that he had learned from the pain that brought him to AA.

"His life had been devastated by alcohol. His geographic cures had included moves to Australia and Mexico, and working in a number of professions. He had alienated his family and had lost two wives and a child. He was living in a house that he owned, renting rooms to other alcoholics, and he looked a little ragged around the edges. He was working at a place that he described as hell. In the face of all of this, he seemed contented and generally happy with where AA was taking him. He talked about wisdom and his ability to sort the bullshit out of any situation or any story.

"When I told him how complex and complicated my thoughts were, he told me to stay away from a drink one day at a time and get to a meeting. When I told him about my fears and apprehensions and my sense of alienation from the world, he told me that for the first year and a half of his sobriety he was convinced he was a Martian and was waiting for the mother ship to snatch him back home. He smiled when he said that. He said that he was familiar with delusions. For a long time while remaining sober, every time he opened his closet, he saw people who weren't there. I asked him how in the hell he adjusted to that. He said he believed the people in the program when they told him that things would pass and he would get better. He gave the phantoms names, and after a while they went away.

"I found strength in his story. I thought to myself, 'If someone that bad can get better, there's hope for me.' When I told him I was losing my profession, my sense of humor, and all of my money, he asked me if I was sober. I said yes I was, and he said that made me a success. No matter what problem I brought to him, his answers were direct and simple and all based on the fundamentals of Alcoholics Anonymous: meditate, pray if you're so inclined, stay away from a drink one day at a time, get to a meeting every day, and things will be all right. If I have gotten anything from the program of Alcoholics Anonymous, it is the absolute certainty that if I live my life according to the program, things will be fundamentally okay with me. They may not be exactly the way I want them to be or the way I think they should be, but they will be fundamentally the way they ought to be."

As time passes, the relationship between sponsor and sponsored becomes more reciprocal. It is impossible to share such intimacy and trust without having the relationship become mutual. The relationship with AA, like sobriety, tends to be cumulative. Members build on the common experience of growth in sobriety and spirituality characteristic of AA involvement. It is often said at meetings and events that once a person gets accustomed to the kind of interaction that goes on in AA, other gatherings become boring or superficial. Among AA members there is little conversation that could pass as chitchat. Subjects not encountered in everyday conversation are the rule.

Note the extent to which the life regimen of the alcoholic is affected by his involvement with AA. He becomes familiar with the literature describing ethical and moral commitments that will ensure appropriate, regulated, and rewarding relationships with other people. He attends at least seven meetings a week where his "disease" is given a dose of AA treatment. A lot of time is taken up in considering the negative impact of alcohol on his life, the nature of his despair, and his lack of fit in the culture. He begins to lessen his isolation. He has, at this time, made a decision about himself. By defining himself an alcoholic, he has explicitly admitted to a need for change. He has been presented with a set of precepts and actions that are guaranteed to bring about the changes necessary to enable him to lead a sober life to good purpose. In being forced to seek out a sponsor and ask that sponsor to help him, he has begun the process of ego deflation. Most importantly, he has admitted his inability to stop drinking on his own and has begun to develop a new sense of why that is. He has begun to recognize that alcoholism is a disease and to define some of his behavior as compulsion generated by alcohol. In his first year, if he works at Steps Four and Five, he begins to develop a new self-image and to like himself again. This is a beginning of self-awareness. Until he forgives himself and bases that forgiveness on understanding, with hope and faith in the possibility of an alcohol-free future, he will never be able to forgive others. Without forgiveness, he will never free himself from the bondage of resentment and isolation. With burgeoning social contacts and an improved self-image, a working relationship with his sponsor, a growing faith in a sober future based on the one-day-at-a-time concept, and daily attendance at meetings, the alcoholic constructs a daily regimen that supports his need for sobriety. It doesn't mean that the path is going to be smooth or unidirectional, moving forward all of the time. It means only that he is laying a foundation on which to build. He learns to manage on a day-to-day basis and to cope with the everyday problems of living sober.

What to Avoid

To sustain sobriety, the alcoholic must be constantly aware of his vulnerability to mind-altering substances. He must keep in mind that he lives in an alcohol- and drug-saturated culture and be aware that alcohol is an ingredient in a large number of products with little or no indication of its presence. Food heads the list of what to look out for. Although it is commonly assumed that all alcohol cooks out of food in preparation, such is not the case. To be on the safe side, the alcoholic is better off not eating food that has been flambéed, poached, or cooked in alcohol, marinated or flavored with alcohol, or had anything at all to do with alcohol. This is not hard to do, but it does require a certain amount of awareness. When dining out it is always a good idea to ask the waiter or waitress if alcohol has been used in the preparation of food, especially desserts. I am not suggesting that if an alcoholic gets a mouthful of dessert that is laced with brandy, he or she will instantly go out and get drunk or suddenly have a compulsion to drink. Mistakes can happen. Good advice: spit it out. Do not feel that the dish must be finished. Alcohol does not belong in an alcoholic's system in any quantity, and it is not safe to take it in any form. Vigilance is the price of sobriety.

The accidental intake of alcohol by an unwary alcoholic at a party or a more formal social function can seem funny. When it happens, it is frightening. Barry described such an incident. "I attended a Christmas party for the staff of a prestigious hospital. There were a number of people there I wanted to meet and wanted to impress. It would be good for my career if they noticed me in a favorable way. I knew that the punch was spiked; the alcohol was on an open bar clearly labeled. I figured out that all of the carafes held wine or wine punch and avoided them. I knew none of the food had been cooked in wine, and my wife had warned me that there was a dark brown cake on the table that the hostess had encouraged her to taste. It was called whiskey cake and had more than a pint of booze in it. My wife said she didn't think it would be a good idea for me to have a slice. I agreed.

"While picking around in the hors d'ouvres, I came upon some brown little balls with a coconut coating. I popped a couple of them in my mouth. I have never been able to resist a carbohydrate. My tongue stood to attention and said, 'Hello there, where have you been so long?' I had been sober more than eight years, but I sure knew that taste. By now I had chewed the two rather large balls into a gummy mass mixed with saliva and other particles of food. I was in a quandary, but the decision was made physically without my being aware of it mentally. The next thing I saw was this big brown blob, looking every bit like doggy doo, falling out of my mouth and landing with a thud on the white tablecloth, just a little left of center on the serving table.

"I didn't have time to turn away and act as if I had nothing to do with it. There was no way I could avoid looking at the mess, and there was no way I could explain to anybody why I stood in front of a table filled with beautifully prepared food and spit a blob of indistinguishable brown mess on it. I have never had more occasion to be grateful that people generally don't want to talk about unpleasant subjects or don't want to recognize something gross even when it happens in front of them. The physical side of my being took over, and I saw myself floating over to the area where the napkins were kept on the table and as calm and as cool as I could be, reaching over and picking up this chewed brown mass, using a knife to scrape the residue from the tablecloth, packing it in the napkins and disappearing into the kitchen. When in the kitchen, I thanked whatever gods there may be for automatic responses.

"For the rest of the evening, I got a few strange looks, but the hostess didn't mention the incident. My wife thought she'd die but sure didn't want me swallowing the stuff. She asked the hostess what those things were. They were bourbon balls. They were made of raw dough similar to brownie dough and copious amounts of bourbon. No wonder my tongue stood to attention. Bourbon had been my drink of choice for years.

"The incident scared me in the sense that I didn't know what would have happened if I had swallowed the mess. I guess the incident frightened me to the extent that I cherish my sobriety. I talked it over with my sponsor. His response was quick and to the point. Mistakes don't count. And then, with an almost winsome look on his face, he said he wished he had been there to watch the projectile land on the table. We were not invited to the next party."

Other Areas of Concern

Other substances to be particularly careful of are mouthwashes, cough medicine, and headache remedies, which frequently contain alcohol. The alcoholic cannot take mood-altering drugs or substances. It is the collective experience of AA that mood-altering drugs of any kind eventually lead to drinking. This is not to suggest that people should abandon medicine prescribed by their doctor without careful consideration. Alcoholics, however, should be aware that tranquilizers are frequently dispensed to calm anxiety, but they have properties that may excite the drive to alter reality. I have heard countless people recount the difficulty in getting off Valium and other prescribed tranquilizers. In some instances, doctors prescribing tranquilizers were not aware of their patient's alcoholism or, if they were aware of it, were not familiar enough with the treatment of alcoholism to realize that the prescription of tranquilizers compounds rather than alleviates alcoholics' problems. Antipsychotic and antidepressant drugs prescribed by physicians as a course of treatment for clinically definable mental illness, are, of course, not included in this discussion. The use of prescribed drugs simply requires careful consideration on the part of the alcoholic and frank discussion with the prescribing physician. It may be good advice to seek a second or even a third opinion.

Almost all commercially available cough medicines and mouthwashes contain alcohol, sometimes in fairly large amounts. I have heard innumerable tales of lapses back into alcoholism that began with getting high from a particular cough medicine, headache remedy (laced with codeine), or mouthwash. In addition to these products, the alcoholic must beware of painkillers of all sorts. These are most frequently prescribed before or after surgery, or after an injury or dental work. The common assumption is that pain is intolerable and that people need to have their senses dulled to endure. For the alcoholic, this is a dangerous proposition. He cannot afford to have his senses dulled and must be aware that there is a relationship between his sensitivity to alcohol and sensitivity to drugs. Many painkillers contain codeine or a narcotic. They are frequently mood altering and have an addictive quality, either physical or psychological.

At a meeting: "I remember when I went into the hospital to have my knee operated on. I had had a motorcycle accident. The knee kept going out of joint, and I kept falling down at the most inappropriate times and in the most inappropriate places. The surgery I was to have was serious but not life threatening. I told the orthopedic surgeon that I was an alcoholic as a part of my physical examination, so he was well aware of my physical dependencies. Preoperatively I found myself having to ward off sleeping pills and injections of tranquilizers. The hospital staff was quite annoyed with me. The norm was that you took the medicine you were given and didn't ask what it was.

"I was finally reduced to taking a stool softener and coated aspirin. Everyone told me how much pain I was going to be in and that it wasn't necessary that I feel a thing. I was told over and over that whatever they would give me would be okay, and I wouldn't be bothered later. It was clear that none of them knew anything about alcoholism or had even bothered to find the word *alcoholic* in my medical chart. I went through the operation with no pre-op shot and woke up in my room. The barrage of people pushing painkillers began in earnest at this point. I refused to take them all despite predictions of dire pain. They were right. I did experience some pain, and I was certainly uncomfortable for a period of time. But my knee healed, and I did not put anything in my system that would reawaken the dragon. Maybe I'm being too careful, I don't know. I just know that the risk of my returning to drinking is too great for me to take any chance at all. I'll stick to the stool softener and aspirin."

Ordinarily, if the alcoholic makes a habit of telling everyone he consults about his physical and mental health that he is an alcoholic, his professional helpers will try to take that into consideration. However, the alcoholic must not assume that the professional with whom he consults will know the consequences to an alcoholic if he takes a mood-altering drug. It is the alcoholic's job to be wary for them both.

Drugs and Alcohol

Recently, there has been a trend of people with dual addictions—that is, people who are alcoholic and involved with other drugs—attending AA meetings. Some of these are people for whom alcohol was the second drug of choice. They prefer AA to Narcotics Anonymous (NA), a program based on Alcoholics Anonymous. With this trend, a new term, *drugging*, has been introduced into the vocabulary of substance abuse. Its most obvious derivation is from the term *drinking*; its invention came about because of the prevalence of mind-altering drugs among young people in the past four or five generations. We are now seeing more polyaddicted patients in treatment facilities and at AA meetings. It is a sad comment on our culture that for the preteen, drugs are much easier to obtain than alcohol. Yet, even given the availability of drugs for the very young, experts agree that alcohol consumption is the major health problem among teenagers and preteens.

Some drug users cease their involvement with drugs when alcohol becomes easily available to them. Alcohol then becomes the drug of choice. The nature of drug addiction, whether psychological or physiological, is not radically different from alcohol addiction. In many cases, the physical damage done by some drugs is less significant than the impact of alcohol on the system.

The addictions differ, however, in the social-psychological context in which they occur and develop. Although there are social rituals that surround drug taking, there are no situations or public rituals associated with drug taking comparable to those involving alcohol. That there is more support for the consumption of alcohol than exists for the taking of drugs would appear to suggest that differences should exist in treatment regimes. Even a cursory look at the relationship between mood-altering drugs and alcohol and how they affect the individual should make it clear that the alcoholic who wants to remain sober cannot take mood-altering drugs of any kind. Not surprisingly, this has been the collective experience of AA members. Almost invariably where the alcoholic substitutes the use of some mild psychogenic drug for alcohol, he returns to the use of alcohol. The relationship of alcohol to those who abuse other substances is probably similar.

It is AA tradition that those primarily addicted to drugs, who identify themselves as drug abusers, may attend meetings but should not share. If called on, they should pass, after identifying themselves by first name. While this tradition is generally understood, it is seldom honored. Both AA and NA have their own literature with differences in approach and emphasis. They do not differ in terms of basic philosophy or infrastructure. In its creation, NA was based on the AA model, adapting the Big Book and existing literature and adding its own literature. In some ways, the NA literature addressing the Steps is more directed and clear. Although it is perfectly permissible to attend either meeting, regardless of addiction type, those chairing AA meetings should reflect allegiance and self-definition.

A young woman, Cindy, was asked to chair an AA meeting by a new meeting secretary. This particular meeting was peopled by a lot of members with long-term sobriety. People here had been to a lot of meetings. They knew how it was supposed to work. As Cindy began to chair and tell her story, difficulties in her presentation became apparent. She was sixteen years old. She described herself as a drug addict, stating that she had decided to switch from NA to AA. After firing her sponsor, she opined that AA meetings were better and larger. She noted that only the language of the two programs was different and that she would learn the "lingo" pretty quickly.

Her story was all about drug use. There was no reference to alcohol. She talked about living with a twenty-year-old boyfriend at twelve years of age. She talked about running away from home time after time, being arrested in crack houses, and finally being arrested and sent to a detox unit by her parents and a court order. She had been sober for six months. Her story of recovery was peppered with her assertions of independence and inability to tolerate being told what to do. All in all, she came across as a willful, headstrong girl, heading for difficulty, virtually untouched by either program. She ended by saying she was back at home living with her parents and attending high school again. During the discussion period, those who responded said they hoped she would be well and would not return to using drugs. Typical of AA, the culture of meetings does not allow for a critical response to what is presented.

When the meeting ended, several women in the program took Cindy aside and in a caring way suggested that she might want to reconsider her commitment to NA. One of the women suggested also that she attend Alateen, which is an offshoot of Al-Anon. She thought that perhaps there Cindy would meet people her own age, with whom she might have more in common. Later, several veteran members suggested to the secretary that he find people to chair meetings who identified themselves as alcoholic and were able to share in such a way that their strength and hope could be of use. There was little doubt that Cindy was in the wrong place and in the wrong role. She was immature and had so little sobriety and so little insight that she had nothing to offer the meeting. It was understood that the meeting benefited her, and she was treated with courtesy. It was, nonetheless, a bump in the road.

As programs addressing addictions have evolved, the lines between them have blurred. One outcome of this is that increasing numbers of dually addicted people are appearing at AA meetings. Listening to their stories, it is impossible to tell what began where. Nonetheless, attendance at both NA and AA meetings usually resolves itself into attendance and allegiance to one or the other. Sometimes the choice follows the evolution of the problem, sometimes not. Sometimes allegiances are chosen based on the social group wherein the majority of the abuse occurred or on the social group or circumstance leading to treatment.

Court Slips

Boundary issues seldom occur, given the nature of meetings and the anarchistic nature of AA's superstructure. They do happen, however. In the mid-1980s, judges in a mid-Atlantic city began sending alcohol-related defendants to AA meetings as a part of plea bargains or sentences. They were required to have meeting attendance verified by representatives at meetings signing slips provided by the court. These persons were typically required to attend three to five meetings per week. Initial AA meeting responses were positive. But as the number of referrals increased and the meetings began to be overwhelmed with numbers of persons attending, perhaps for the wrong reasons, resistance developed. Throughout the city meetings began resisting signing court slips. Court slips were always a part of meetings, but referrals to AA had never been institutionalized nor sent in these numbers.

The behavior of those assigned to AA was sometimes inappropriate, and meetings began to be overwhelmed by them. They would sit in the back of meetings, talking among themselves, reading newspapers, drinking coffee, but never contributing to the meetings themselves. They just came to get their court slips signed. As hostility among traditional AA attendees grew, meetings began to refuse to sign court slips. Memberships at meetings held group conscience meetings and found themselves split as to whether or not to sign. Those opposed to signing were reminded of AA's early history, wherein membership numbers were drawn from courts assigning alcoholics to Dr. Bob's care in his role as a medical doctor.

New meetings were formed over the issues. Resentments over the directions meetings took frequently lead to the creation of new meetings: "All you need is a coffee pot and resentment." There were directives from the general office in New York, and slip signing was not recommended. The general feeling was that AA should not keep track of alcoholics for the court. After a while, the problem seemed to fix itself. Slips were no longer signed as a matter of policy, and the courts stopped the blanket referrals. Selective referrals to AA have resulted in certain meetings signing courts slips again—yet another bump in the road. Because AA's leadership and policies avoid taking positions on virtually anything, time and normal attrition seem to settle most struggles. As was said recently at a group conscience meeting (a meeting at which people officially designated as members of a group meet to discuss issues), meetings just seem to persist; "the dogs bark but the caravan moves on."

Prayer

The act of prayer is another mechanical aid to achieving sobriety. It is no accident that the literature of AA suggests prayer and/or meditation as an aid to sobriety. Their importance is emphasized frequently in meetings as well. The AA membership contains a wide range of religious and spiritual beliefs, so the choice of meditation or prayer as a daily part of a program of sobriety is personal. One can do both. The two are not mutually exclusive. For the alcoholic who has no traditional belief in God or need to have one, meditation can be undertaken as a discipline but prayer is a remote possibility at best. There is a way to reconcile prayer with agnosticism, thereby providing yet another tool on which to build the sober life. After all, membership in AA begins with the promise to "go to any lengths" to achieve sobriety.

How can the agnostic pray without slipping into hypocrisy? AA members are told over and over again that the program must be based on honesty or it will fail. How can the agnostic hold that there is no phone on the other end of the line of prayer? Certainly, it depends on how one conceives of prayer. The impact of prayer on sobriety depends on the content of the prayer and not on its reception. If one is convinced that there is no God, then prayer is a statement of intent, wish, or condition. Members are often told to be careful what they pray for because they might get it. The importance of prayer and its impact increase as the content of prayer becomes less self-centered and is directed more toward others.

Jim R. comments, "One of the most difficult things that I had to work on in the development of my program in AA was resentment. There were people I just couldn't stand, and I resented them. There were circumstances in my life that were so painful to me that I resented them and everyone connected with them. I had a neighbor who was particularly intrusive, and I resented her beyond measure. She complained to me constantly about everything from pine needles from my trees blowing into her yard, to my dog's barking, to my children crying in the night, to where I parked my car. She threw branches over the fence separating our properties and vandalized my car. Every time I saw her, I saw red and seethed inside. When we spoke to one another, it was for her to complain and for me to tell her to go straight to hell without bothering to shut the door. The woman was a thorn in my side and caused me disruption on a daily basis.

"I talked about her at meetings, and my sponsor told me that I had to do something to resolve this situation because it was interfering with my working the Steps. My sponsor finally told me that I had better start praying for the woman and trying to have good thoughts about her. I was cautioned again that the alcoholic could not afford anger, much less self-righteous anger, and that resentment frequently led to drinking. I told my sponsor that I didn't believe in prayer and that I was an agnostic. I was, however, comfortable with the notion of a higher power.

"I didn't pray for myself or for other members of the family. I considered prayer to be kind of emotional-philosophical masturbation, momentarily satisfying but in the end leading nowhere. My sponsor suggested that I had more to worry about than just resentment. He felt that I had ego problems to deal with and that I should begin to think about my arrogance. He cautioned me against closing my mind to possibilities, suggesting that there might be something in the technique of prayer itself that could help me in my program of sobriety. He reminded me of my beginnings in AA and again told me that it wasn't necessary that I understand what was going on; it was only necessary that I do what I was told.

"I began a kind of prayer for my neighbor that very evening. I began my prayer with 'to whomever it may concern or whatever there is or isn't out there in the universe.' I always ended by feeling a little foolish. At first I prayed for her demise. Then, I began praying that she find some way of minding her own business. A little later on I found myself praying that she find a way of not letting things annoy her the way they did. A little further down the line, I found myself genuinely praying that she be comfortable. The more my prayers were directed to good things and serenity for her, the better I began to feel.

"Much to my surprise, I lost my feelings of resentment toward her. She hasn't changed at all. I have changed in my reaction to her. I don't feel badly when I see her, and I am no longer angry at her. To the contrary, I find myself understanding her and still wishing that good things happen to her. I was both surprised and somewhat appalled at this turn of events, and I used the technique to help me get over other resentments. It works. I remain an agnostic, but I am convinced that prayer, as a simple activity, regardless of the mysteries that exist in the world, is good to the extent that its content is selfless."

The content of prayer evidently affects its impact on sobriety and at the same time acts as a barometer or benchmark for other elements of growth in the program. Below is a short list of types of prayer and what they represent to the development of an AA program. Please keep in mind that the list is not meant to be exhaustive.

1. Selfless prayers to help others. Prayers of this type can aid in the abatement of resentment and other negative forms of thinking that are pernicious to sobriety, as well as provide a general upbeat tone for any given day. The healthy alcoholic bases his relationship with others on a noncontrolling, non-ego-oriented basis.

2. Thy will be done. These prayers, which characteristically seek direction for living along ethical and moral lines, are generally helpful to the alcoholic. Keep in mind that we have in many ways defined the alcoholic as suffering from a case of "self-will run riot." Prayers of this type seek a life based on ethical and moral precepts that guarantee a smooth passage through life. The offerer of this prayer isn't fighting things or people anymore. He is not trying to change the world to suit his needs. To the contrary, he is controlling the only thing he can control, himself and his feelings. This type of prayer also crystallizes the alcoholic's surrender to his alcoholism. He knows that his sobriety is not a function of willpower but rather involves identification with a collective purpose in AA and a collective solution to his dilemma.

3. Keep me sober. Prayers of this variety also recognize surrender. In addition, they seek help and recognition of the futility of isolated struggles. Solutions lie in the experience of the group.

4. Help me be patient, help me be honest, and so on. Prayers that seek help with specific tasks sharpen the focus of the individual's efforts and provide checklists for the daily inventories suggested as a measure of personal growth in sobriety.

5. Prayer of thanks. These prayers are particularly important because they help remind the alcoholic that he is not solely responsible for his sobriety. He has exercised a discipline, but the solution to his alcoholism was a collective one derived from the moral and ethical experience of past and present members. His thanks remind him of his responsibility to service in the program to help other suffering alcoholics.

Prayer is no hypocrisy for the agnostic or the atheist if it is seen as affecting that individual's activity rather than as asking for a "good" that depends on the prayer's being answered by someone or something.

Meditation is easy for the religiously committed and the uncommitted to accept as a practice. A simple definition of meditation is a period of quiet time during the day. It is a time to empty the mind by focusing on a single object or sound and to let the mind drain and be at peace. This is not the time to think about problems or tasks. Meditation is quiet time uncluttered by external concerns. Mindfulness is another form of meditation where thoughts are observed and allowed to move through the consciousness without the mind dwelling on any one thought. Rather, one observes the thought and allows it to pass without focusing on it, worrying about it, or judging it. It is a method of increasing self-awareness and skill in living in the present.

Slogans

Among the most annoying and obvious tools AA uses to aid sobriety are the various slogans that festoon the walls and tables of meeting rooms all over the world. They are a collection of bromides, hopeful homilies, and statements of the obvious, carefully calligraphed, framed, and lovingly displayed. They are seen by all newcomers, quoted by a sober membership, and peppered throughout the literature. If any single element of the program is universally despised by newcomers, it is the slogans. Despite their commonsense wisdom, they almost always become important to virtually all who stay in Alcoholics Anonymous for a reasonable period of time. Here are just a few of them:

1. But for the grace of God
2. Think
3. One day at a time
4. Keep coming back
5. KISS (keep it simple, stupid)
6. Journeys begin with one step
7. HALT (do not allow yourself to become Hungry, Angry, Lonely, or Tired)

Each of the slogans is meant to bolster attitudes that are perceived to be important in maintaining sobriety. "But for the grace of God" reminds alcoholics that they are fortunate to be in a place where they can find help. As a matter of simple probability they could be floundering, unable or unwilling to seek help, and condemned to living the alcoholic life. The admonition, "THINK" is self-explanatory. The content of that thought process, by implication, is the program of Alcoholics Anonymous. It cautions alcoholics to think before they act. They are frequently told to let twenty-four hours pass before they react to any situation. It is always good advice. The word *think* is an admonition not to be impulsive but to consider each action carefully and to weigh it against the moral and ethical instructions of the AA program.

"One day at a time" is a particularly important concept for alcoholics. In the program, people do not give up drinking forever. They simply forestall that drink. They stop drinking one day at a time. In the beginning they may very well stop drinking one hour at a time or one half-hour at a time or in some cases one minute at a time. The important thing is that they can do things for a twenty-four-hour period that they couldn't conceive of doing over a lifetime. One hears "one day at a time" as the subject of many meetings, and for a large number of alcoholics it is the single most important concept in their first year of sobriety.

"Keep coming back." This phrase is probably used more in Alcoholics Anonymous than any other, and it is the most frequently heard by newcomers. Regardless of their complaint, be it physical, psychological or social, they are cautioned to stay away from a drink, one day at a time, and to keep coming back. The solution offered to any and all problems for the newcomer is keep coming back. AA must be the centerpiece of the alcoholic's life if he is to get sober. All things flow from that. He will most frequently be told that if he doesn't put AA first he won't have to worry about what will be second or third in his life. This is another way of saying that for the newcomer the most important part of his developing program of sobriety is daily attendance at meetings. There is no substitute for this regardless of what happens. The alcoholic must stay away from a drink one day at a time and keep coming back.

"Keep it simple, stupid" is another phrase of signal importance to the newcomer. Some of the older heads in the program prefer the phrase, "Keep it simple, sweetheart." People are in the program because they are alcoholics and not because they are stupid. The phrase was borrowed from the profession of engineering, where it is commonly used regarding design. Whether one uses *stupid* or *sweetheart,* the admonition is clear. In order for a program of sobriety to be effective, it must be simple in content and simple in application. The process of getting sober in Alcoholics Anonymous is not complicated and does not require overinterpretation. It requires cooperation and daily discipline, but it is exceedingly easy to understand. It is not necessarily easy to analyze with regard to its impact or effectiveness. It is simply easy to work.

The phrase "Journeys begin with one step" is particularly aimed at newcomers, although it pertains to old-timers as well. Goals are achieved by increments and not by leaps. For the newcomer, the prospect of stopping drinking and interrupting lifetime patterns of alcoholic behavior may seem daunting. It is wise to remind oneself that all journeys begin with one step. For the alcoholic, that one step is surrender.

For the alcoholic, "HALT" is also good advice. It tells alcoholics not to get too hungry, too angry, too lonely, or too tired if they are to maintain sobriety. It is, if you will, an admonition to do all things in moderation and avoid excesses. Decisions made while experiencing a physical and/or psychological imbalance are usually bad decisions.

At meetings one hears about the slogans all the time. At one meeting, a particularly striking woman sitting at the rear of the group was called on to share. She gave her name and said that she had a problem with alcohol and had come to the meeting to see whether AA had anything to offer her and whether she was willing to participate in it. She was haughty, even arrogant, and openly questioned whether or not the group would come up to her standards. People at the meeting told her to keep coming back. I saw the same woman at a meeting about a year later. She was chairing. A part of her story included a description of her first night at AA. She talked about how frightened she felt and how arrogant she had been in expecting AA to audition for her.

"When I looked around the room at the meetings that I attended, I saw little signs tacked up everywhere. They were corny and short. I thought to myself that it was good that they were there because they were probably all that these people could handle. I knew I was superior to everyone in the room, and I knew that the slogans were there to help other people. I was capable of significantly more analysis and was sure that my program of recovery would be at a much higher plane. I made up my mind to tolerate the slogans and the people. In spite of this, I stayed sober.

"After a while, I found myself thinking the slogans. At first I didn't notice it, but after a while I couldn't deny it. I would be having a lousy time, and I would think, 'this too shall pass.' When I thought about drinking, I thought I could stay away from it 'one day at a time.' I began telling newcomers 'to keep coming back.' I don't know how it happened, but one by one I owned the slogans. I had so much fun with what I had resented when I came into AA."

8. Easy does it
9. Remember when
10. Live and let live
11. Principles above personalities

Of all the slogans in AA, "Easy does it" is perhaps the most used and the most abused. It instructs the alcoholic to go a little easy on himself, not to push so hard, and to let time bind up troubles and wounds. It is a way of suggesting that sobriety requires a kind of gentleness of mind and spirit in order that healing take place. It is a caution against rushing pell-mell into decisions that may be regretted later. The slogan, however, has been used to justify outright laziness, with "easy does it" being the passport to sitting around and doing nothing. Some in the program have added "but do it" to the slogan. The slogan has even been made into a bumper sticker.

The slogan "Remember when" is self-explanatory. Alcoholics attend meetings so that they do not forget the circumstances that brought them to AA and their surrender to alcoholism in the first place.

"Live and let live" is another one of those expressions that has been put on bumper stickers. In AA it is interpreted to mean not only exhibiting tolerance but living that tolerance without the condescension that normally accompanies it. Another AA interpretation of "live and let live" has to do with Step Four, the inventory Step. It cautions AA members not to take the inventory of others. It's a standing joke in AA that, of all the Steps, you can get the greatest amount of help with Step Four. This is true both in and out of AA. People are always willing to tell you what's wrong with you but less willing to consider what's wrong with them.

Rusty B. was recently talking about the importance of the slogans at a meeting. "I was sober about a year and a half, and thought I was working a pretty good program. I went to seven or eight meetings a week and enjoyed them. I developed a bunch of friends in AA that met at meetings. All in all I felt pretty secure. My service to AA consisted of putting chairs away from time to time and talking about being a power of example. Although I wasn't asked to chair very many meetings and didn't share very often when called on at a meeting, I had a lot to say about what other people shared and what their chances of staying sober were. I made personal comments about one and all. This had been somewhat of a pattern with me, and I assumed that everyone did it. All I was doing was listening to me.

"One evening, about twenty minutes before the meeting was finished, I was giving a run down on what I thought the chances were of a couple of people who had just begun coming to our group. A young woman tapped me on the shoulder, got my attention, and pointed to a sign on the wall that said 'Live and let live.' I joked about that too but began to wonder what she was trying to tell me. It took a couple of hours of thinking and my sponsor to explain to me what was wrong with taking other people's inventory and how many of my attitudes reflected my intolerance and indifference.

"It took a long while for me to stop taking the inventory of other people and to focus on what was wrong with me. When I really began working on my own inventory, I found that I had more than enough to keep me busy. I didn't need to worry about other people. Probably the most important lesson I learned from all this was how to give other people room to live around me. I am not as judgmental as I used to be, and I am willing to assume that when people disappoint me they are generally doing the very best that they can. It is hard to be angry with people when you assume they are doing about the best they can. I don't know what all these corny slogans have done for other people, but they have been a regular reminder to me of my own frailty and my own need for change and growth in AA. At first I didn't pay any attention to them. Now I point them out to other people."

"Principles above personalities" is a slogan derived directly from the Traditions of Alcoholics Anonymous. It simply means don't confuse the message with the messenger. As Rusty says, "In AA you meet a lot of people, some of whom are not going to be your exact cup of tea. It is important to remember that you can learn from the experience and that it isn't necessary that you like everyone you meet in AA. It is necessary that you love them, but it isn't necessary that you like them."

The slogans are short, to the point, and easy to remember. They are posted everywhere in meeting rooms and are an excellent way of remembering some of the basic principles of Alcoholics Anonymous. The slogans are effective because they are about principles. They caution alcoholics to be grateful for their sobriety, to think about actions before they leap into them, to control their anger, and to try to develop and grow one day at a time. The importance of meetings is stressed, as well as the essential simplicity of the program that guarantees to keep alcoholics sober. They are told to care for themselves psychologically as well as physically, to do things at a steady comfortable pace, and to remember their past so that they do not have to repeat it. It is important to be courteous and understanding of other people, keeping in mind that they bring limitations to life just as everyone does, and that the message is more important then the messenger. Perhaps the unifying concept in all the slogans is that annoying principle we talked about earlier. When we have trouble with others or other things, the trouble lies within ourselves.

Being Involved

Recall that the organization of Alcoholics Anonymous was founded on a single discovery. When Bill W. discovered that the key to his own sobriety was trying to help another alcoholic get sober, the seeds of AA were sown. Indeed, helping other alcoholics understand their plight and showing them a method of achieving sobriety through the use of one's own experiences and struggles constitute a cornerstone of Alcoholics Anonymous. It is often suggested that identification with AA as an organization and a program of recovery really begins with involvement at various levels of service.

To understand the importance of involvement, consider the broad range of services offered at no cost through AA. Alcoholics have at their fingertips unlimited therapy sessions taking place in various parts of the city throughout the day and night, twenty-four-hour-a-day phone lines where immediate help is available, unlimited time with counselors (sponsors) and others offering support in the struggle against alcohol, a worldwide network of meetings and literature, a panorama of social and educational activities, and complete coordination of recovery services. All of this is provided by an organization that charges no fees or dues. Obviously, the service of its members is an important element in its ongoing progress. When new to AA, individual service can be helping to set up chairs, making coffee, or cleaning up after a meeting. For many, these small tasks are things they have not done before or that they have defined as being "beneath them." It is good to be useful, and performing such service is good for the ego as well. Ben B., a well-to-do business entrepreneur, described his beginning services at AA.

"I had been sober six months, and my sponsor asked me to help with a meeting. It was what we call a high-bottom meeting; that is, it was being held at a prestigious church in a beautiful room. Members who frequented this particular meeting were residents of the surrounding expensive suburb and were given to intellectualizing alcoholism and the achievement of almost hourly insights. Later in my sobriety I came to prefer a more 'guts and thunder' type of meeting, but the intellectual gloss of this meeting appealed to me in early sobriety. When I was asked to help with the meeting, I thought my sponsor wanted me to run it. Instead, he asked me to put away a few chairs after the meeting and help wash ashtrays. I got sore as hell, although I didn't tell him about it.

"I offered to have one of the people who worked for me do the setup and come in afterward to clean up. In fact, I offered to have the meeting catered. I said that way we could spend more time getting sober and talking about AA. As I warmed to the idea, I told him that I could define this as a business expense and that it would be a way for me to show my gratitude to the group for my sobriety. My sponsor didn't say much. He showed me where the towels were and where to stack the ashtrays.

"I began to get a sense of what was wrong with me soon after that. I bitched, but I did what I was told. I started to get a handle on humility. I didn't realize just how total my changes were going to have to be. I couldn't buy any part of it. I was going to have to pitch in and do a lot of things that I thought were beneath my dignity. More importantly, I was going to have to begin relating to my sobriety in terms other than my own. Prior to my getting sober, my external achievements were what I held on to as a way of showing my self-worth. In AA, other qualities were valued. I came to define these internal measures as the yardstick of my success as a person. No one was impressed with my money or my business success. As much as I wanted to impress them, they kept telling me that I didn't like myself very much.

"My service in AA began with putting away chairs and washing ashtrays. In the ensuing years I have been the secretary of a meeting, and I have been privileged to serve on various state and national boards affecting AA policy in general. I have never forgotten the lesson, however, that any service in AA is of value to my sobriety and that service of all kinds is equally valuable. It has been a long while since I have been impressed with my own self-importance. I don't want to be 'Mr. AA,' nor do I want recognition for my work in AA. My reward is AA; it has been ample. My reward has been my own sobriety."

Vigilance and a willingness to change serve to protect sobriety. Equally important are self-awareness and participation in a social system that supports your identity as a sober person. It is as important to remember where you came from as it is to know where you are going.

7

THE ALCOHOLIC AND THE FAMILY

Alcoholism is a family disease. Every member of the alcoholic's nuclear and extended family is affected by it. The social and financial aspects of family life are clearly damaged, and alcoholism frequently generates legal (criminal and civil) problems. Other effects are more subtle but nonetheless devastating. They derive from the nature of the impact of alcohol on the alcoholic. They derive from the furtiveness, self-centeredness, fundamental dishonesty, obsession, erratic social behavior, and isolation that attend being alcoholic. It is sad but true that alcoholics will do virtually anything in their power to change the direction or the quality of their lives, except stop drinking.

The alcoholic is frequently aided in denial and the continuation of drinking by friends and family who insist that while the person drinks too much, he or she "isn't an alcoholic." It is as if the family and friends in admitting the alcoholism of one of its members shares in the shame. The term *alcoholic* denotes shame enough for all. It is a social disgrace to be married to an alcoholic as well as to parent an alcoholic child. In both instances, either judgment, choice, or the effectiveness of parenting are questioned. In the very act of denial and, more commonly, in the name of support in times of trouble, families enable the alcoholic to continue drinking. Enabling is the process of standing between alcoholics and the consequences of their drinking. Wayne Z. describes his family at an Al-Anon meeting.

"Alcohol did a job on me. I flunked out of college, lied to my family by telling them that I had quit out of disinterest. I took a job with an individual whom I had worked for during the summer. He was an alcoholic. He and I worked together and drank together. He was the president and owner of a corporation, and I was his favorite son. By the time I was twenty-eight years old, I had an unlimited expense account, a new car provided every year by the company, I made my own hours and in general did what I pleased. No amount of abuse could lose me my job. I took care of that problem; I quit. I told my employer that I couldn't take any more of his bullshit and walked away. He told me I was crazy. He was my first real enabler.

"My family enabled me to drink throughout high school and my first year of college, chalking my erratic and antisocial behavior up to the high jinks of youth. I don't think they have come to grips even today with my alcoholism. After I quit my job, I lived on savings and took a year off. When I began to look for work, I found that I wasn't willing to accept any imposition on my freedom or my time. Naturally, I bought a bar. I sank every penny of my savings into the venture. It took two years to drink my way through a successful business, turning it, too, into a failure.

"Throughout this, my friends told me that I needed to get myself together. I recall vividly that at one point I told the people I was in business with that I had to stop drinking, that I felt I was an alcoholic. They told me that I worked too many hours and that probably what I needed to do was slow down a little. When the business failed because of my poor judgment and lack of attention, no one blamed my drinking. I was physically and spiritually exhausted and as isolated as I could be. I was afraid of my own shadow. I was out of money and had nothing left to sell.

"I moved to Florida to stay with an aunt who had partly raised me. I cleaned houses for her to make a modest living. I stayed with her rent-free. Her condition for my staying included that I stop drinking. I hid liquor all over the house. She found wine bottles under the bed. I felt like a teenager, but I couldn't stop drinking. No matter how many times I broke the rules, she did not throw me out of the house. When I ran out of money, she gave it to me. She seemed to feel that this was the only way to help me. In a sense, she did help: she helped me postpone my bottom. I didn't hit bottom until I left her house and tried to make it again on my own. I was thrown out of my apartment, and my car was repossessed. I found myself on the street with empty pockets, with a bad wine habit, and so isolated that I had nowhere to turn. I applied for welfare and was referred to a mission.

"I heard about AA at the mission. I knew of AA before, but I always felt that my problems stemmed from sources other than drinking. I felt that drinking was the only thing that helped me through my life. I attended an AA meeting, and I heard my story. I was so devastated by everything that had happened to me and so spiritually and emotionally dead that I latched on to

AA. I thought at least it could help me feel better and maybe it could help me get a job.

"I have been sober for a number of years, and my life has turned around. Incredibly, many of the people who enabled me throughout my drinking career are still unable to confront the fact of my alcoholism. They talk about my nervous breakdown and hospitalization and ask all the time why I go to meetings so frequently, suggesting that I don't need them. 'After all, you've been sober for quite a while.' I don't explain anything to them. I didn't get sober for them. I got sober for myself. It wasn't easy."

How difficult it is for people surrounding the alcoholic to care about him yet to separate love from responsibility. How difficult it is to know what to do in the long run. For this reason, families take care of immediate needs and contingencies, and alcoholics are protected from the consequence of drinking. The wife who calls the husband "in sick" and lies to the boss about why he is missing work is an enabler. The children who make excuses for parental absences at school functions are enablers. The people who pay bills for alcoholics and supply them with a daily allowance when they are out of work are enablers. In most instances, they do what they do out of concern and love, with little thought given to the long-range effect of standing between the alcoholic and the results of drinking. So much harm is done in the name of love.

Love and the Alcoholic

At times, the most pernicious thing for alcoholics is love. They perceive its loss, mourn its passing, cheapen it with manipulation, chase it in bars, feed fantasy with alcoholic delusions, and cannot give it up because of their obsession with self. Frequently, they perceive themselves as unloved (with good reason—drunks are not loveable). If they see themselves as loved, it's by the wrong people. Mostly, they don't love themselves. They use the love of others to serve the needs of their drinking. Love won't get them sober, and love won't keep them sober. It is in the nature of alcohol and its effects on alcoholics that they do not perceive genuine emotion. What emotions they do feel are exaggerated and pertain to what they want and are not getting. Alcoholics have a classic selfish love affair with themselves. In sobriety, a benchmark of progress is change in attitudes toward the family. In sobriety, love for family and others should become more selfless and less manipulative. Untreated, the alcoholic spends his time serving his addiction. He is self-willed, selfish, obsessed with alcohol, and manipulative, with a drive to control the scene around him. Obviously, such a person is difficult to live with. Because alcohol's effects can be unpredictable, the alcoholic's personality is mercurial and his behavior is erratic. It is easier to trigger a negative response in an alcoholic than in people who don't drink. People around him simply don't know what's coming next or how to react.

As the alcoholism reaches its middle and later stages, it is more and more an unshareable problem. It becomes the center of serious marital conflict and furtive behavior. In such a circumstance, the spouse begins to play the role of warden and conscience. He or she reasons, complains, consoles, begs, and cries. "Stop drinking, slow down. Why do you do this to yourself? Think of the children." It is not that alcoholics don't care for their families. It is just that they don't see alcohol as related to any of the problems they are experiencing.

The alcoholic husband complains that his wife isn't what she used to be. She doesn't understand. Children constitute an intrusion and a responsibility. Wife and children become reasons or excuses for drinking. Like the other excuses for drinking, these are rationalizations rather than causes. The more the wife plays the role of conscience and insists on his stopping drinking, the more she is resented. It is a characteristic of the alcoholic that he resents or avoids anything that gets between him and his drinking. Given a choice between family and the bottle, the alcoholic will usually choose the bottle. He may make stabs at stopping for a while, but the cures he seeks are intended to be temporary. When discussing sobriety, he is planning when he can drink again. Typically, as an aspect of the wife's denial, she is willing to believe that her husband may have a drinking problem but that the problem can be solved by exercising willpower and "only having a couple once in a while." What we see in operation here is the old "yeah, he drinks too much but he isn't that bad" syndrome. Perhaps the wife is afraid to admit that she is married to an alcoholic, either because of the stigma or the bleak future that the term *alcoholic* portends for the family.

Brooks T. discussed this problem at a meeting that focused on the role of the family. "I was married fresh out of college. My wife knew that I drank, but she didn't know how much. In fact, nobody knew how much I drank, and I did my best to stay confused enough so that I didn't know how much I drank.

For me, drinking was a daily activity. It had been part of my college career, and in fact it had taken me five years to finish four years' worth of courses. I was popular in my fraternity and had been elected president of the senior class. My platform was that I wouldn't do anything at all and would therefore be a benign representative. On this basis, I was elected. I had the reputation of being a happy-go-lucky type, and my wife seemed to like that.

"I went into sales and playing house. The first thing I bought was a bar and liquor cabinet combination for the dining room. We had that before we had rugs on the floor or a bed. I was a pretty good salesman, and my wife worked full time. We had more money than we ever had before. I began to drink in earnest. I don't mean that I planned or thought about drinking in earnest. I mean that conditions and circumstances just seemed to provide me with the opportunity of drinking whenever I wanted to. I wasn't concerned about my drinking, so I didn't think it unusual that I seemed to be drinking all day.

"Because I was a salesman, my time was my own, and my circumstances were virtually unsupervised. My wife and I seemed to spend less and less time together. It was partly because we both worked and that I was out in the evenings, but it was more than that. There was something fundamentally going wrong with our relationship. I realize now that it was alcohol. It's crazy, but long before she started complaining about my drinking and asking me if I didn't think I drank too much, I was hiding alcohol in the house and in the car and hiding the amount that I drank from her. As a matter of fact, I didn't drink around her.

As my need increased, this became increasingly difficult. As drinking began to take over my life, I became grateful for the times of separation. On the weekends she filled her Saturdays with errands that involved me less and less. My day was occupied. I drank. I don't mean I got drunk in the falling-down sense of the word. I mean that I drank until I took a nap (translate: passed out) and then would wake up refreshed and drink some more until I got sleepy again. The day was spent in a gentle phasing in and out of life.

"I resented her coming home. After a while, we were spending much of the time fighting when we were together. It just wasn't worth it. The subject was invariably my drinking, and the arguments were always directed toward what she didn't do for me, what was wrong with the world, the screwing I was getting on my job, that I worked hard, and that I wasn't drinking too much anyway. All of my denial mechanisms were in place. In fact, I wasn't working very hard. I seldom saw more than one or two clients a day, and then I tried to take them out to lunch so that I could continue drinking. I spent a lot of time in bars during the day plotting and planning what I was going to do to-morrow to pull my flagging career together.

"As time went by, my wife became more and more determined to stamp out my drinking. The perfunctory kiss in the morning and in the evening as I came and went was a breath test to see whether or not I had been drinking. If she smelled 'Sen-Sen' or any lozenge-type breath deodorants, she raised holy hell with me. The assumption was that if my breath smelled minty, I was drinking. So I brushed my teeth all the time. I had the cleanest teeth in town.

"After a while, she didn't bother checking. She just knew I had been drink-ing. She searched the house for booze, and when she found the bottle that I had hidden, I would be confronted with it. I, of course, denied that I had ever seen it before. It made sense to me. The more she complained, the less I was impressed. The more often she threatened to leave, the more I began to like the idea. I could look at her and feel love for her and yet when forced to make a decision between her and the alcohol, I picked alcohol every time.

"She suspected for a long while that I had a cache of booze hidden in the basement. She never did find out where it was. It was hidden in the insulation in the drop ceiling. She didn't bother taking that apart. But I developed the habit of going down the stairs backwards so that it always looked as if I was coming out of the basement rather then going into it. I reasoned that she would not think that I was going down into the basement to drink but was coming out of the basement after doing something useful. Why I did not imagine that she would have thought I was coming up out of the basement after drinking I do not know. In spite of fuzzy logic this was my practice.

"I eventually fell down the stairs, breaking my leg. My wife was cold to-ward me and unsympathetic. I really resented this. Things finally came to a head when my wife said that she wanted to take a trip to the islands with some girlfriends. She said she needed some time to rest. I thought it was a wonder-ful idea. It would give me at least a week of unsupervised activity in the house. After she had gone a few days, during which time I just stayed at home and drank, she called and told me that she didn't expect that she would be return-ing to the house and that she would send some friends for her clothes.

"Our marriage was finished, and I didn't feel all that badly about it. I felt as if a major impediment to me doing what I wanted to do had been removed. Our finances had been in chaos when she left because I did bills. When they came in the mail, I put them into the desk drawer and closed and locked it.

I ignored all of my responsibilities. I wasn't earning any money. I couldn't pay the bills anyway so why open them and let the amount bother me? My car went, the house went, and finally I went.

The job went, and I moved back in with my mother. She began complaining about my drinking. I ended up in a hospital and finally ended up here in AA. It's difficult for me to assess the damage I did to my wife or how much she helped me in my drinking because she loved me. When I tried to make amends to her, she was gentle with me but told me that she had finally decided to leave me because of the anxiety that my drinking created combined with her unwillingness to stand by and watch me kill myself. She didn't believe that she could ever trust me again. More importantly, she felt that alcoholics never recover and that the rest of her life was not going to be lived in a sewer. She wasn't up to that at all. She wanted to make me feel better about what had happened, but sober I could see the pain and all of its long-range residuals. I wished her a happy life."

Brooks's wife protected him from the consequence of his drinking. She confronted him but offered no help, alternatives, or consequences. She could not stop drinking for Brooks, but she could have tried to understand the process of his disease. In the end she helped. Her leaving precipitated the downward spiral until Brooks hit bottom and sought help. She could have led a better life had she known how to separate from Brooks's alcoholism.

Being the wife of an alcoholic is no bed of roses. It seems as if nothing the wife does is right. Being the husband of an alcoholic is equally difficult. The enabling process, however, takes on a different form. Characteristically, it involves assuming control of children and assuming major responsibility for keeping a house functioning. The female alcoholic who stays at home and does her drinking there is perhaps the most isolated and most dependent of all. Social controls and consequences are fewer. Remember that the dependency on alcohol is the same in all of these cases. The impact of alcoholism is the same. Only the external circumstances of drinking vary.

In many ways, the circumstances surrounding the drinking career of the alcoholic are dictated by the social role that he or she plays. Maleness or femaleness does not appear to have any impact on the essential nature of alcoholism but is reflected in the external circumstances surrounding drinking patterns. This is true of the enabling process also. Husbands enable wives to drink and protect them from the consequences of their drinking differently than wives protect husbands. The end result is the same. In acting in a protective role toward his wife, the husband acts out a traditional and approved role. Men are supposed to protect the women they love. The consequences of protection are often contrary to intentions.

Paul B., a tall, dignified man in his mid-fifties, addressed an Al-Anon meeting. As a physician, he had worked in a metropolitan area all his life. His two children had gone to college and were leading their own lives. At present he lives alone. He had been married to a practicing alcoholic for twenty-seven years. His wife died a year ago from alcoholism complicated by drug abuse. He continued his long membership in Al-Anon to share his story and hope with others. He said Al-Anon had made his life livable. When he began to speak, you could sense that this was a man who had made peace with himself. He had remained an enabler to his wife, however, up until the time of her death.

"Jean's drinking didn't become a problem until the kids were in high school. I never saw her drink. She acted funny once in a while when the kids were small but not often. She frequently took naps in the afternoon and after the kids were in high school began neglecting simple tasks around the house. She frequently neglected to cook dinner. Then she seemed to make a complete turnaround and would clean like crazy and cook elaborate meals. We didn't talk much about it, but she became increasingly difficult to predict. The periods of her overconcern with the house and with the meals became less and less frequent. I started to find wine bottles in strange places. I found two of them in the toilet tank, for example. When I asked her what they were dong there, she said she kept them cool there. Pills started disappearing from my bag and desk.

For the next several years, things stayed about the same. Jean's drunkenness wasn't obvious to anyone but her family. When she got pills, she took them and just went to bed. After a while, her lack of involvement in the family seemed the way it should be. In the beginning, I fought, argued, and complained. I extracted promises I knew she would never keep. At the same time, I provided money and a home and didn't do anything to restrict her. The kids learned to fend for themselves, and I ate out.

"Life went on. I tried to get help for Jean, but she wouldn't go to AA or see a doctor. She kept insisting that she didn't have a problem. She was fiercely protective of her drinking and flew into rages at any suggestion that she drank too much or that she was drunk. When she was sober, she was remorseful about her behavior but not overtly so. She showed her sorrow in her frequent attempts to stop drinking and during the periods when she was successful in moderating her drinking at least to the point where her involvement with family increased.

"I joined Al-Anon. The kids found outside interests. Once in a while they attended Al-Anon meetings. They loved their mother but couldn't control her. I got closer to the kids, and we hired a lady to come in and clean. I got more and more detached from Jean's drinking. I honestly don't know if I would have left her if I had been in another religion. I probably would have.

"The further Jean got into her alcoholism and her pill abuse, the more I guarded my samples and kept suggesting AA. Jean wouldn't go. She continued to stop drinking from time to time, but as time went on she had less and less luck with it. I found myself more detached from her as well as from her drinking. I enjoyed the kids, and life just went on. When Jean died, I found that I still loved her and missed her, but to be honest, I was also relieved. Liver disease was the official cause for her death, but it was alcohol that killed her. She was forty-eight when she died. To this day, I don't know why she couldn't face her disease or get help with it, but she just couldn't."

Not all stories in AA and Al-Anon have a happy ending. For all of his involvement in Al-Anon, Paul kept enabling his wife to drink. He got just enough from Al-Anon to be comfortable himself but not enough to be of help to his wife. Perhaps he would not have been helpful if he had tried to leave his wife or force the issue with an intervention; perhaps she would have continued to drink. On the other hand, perhaps faced with the absolute consequence of her drinking, she would have sought help. We will never know.

Al-Anon

The Al-Anon movement began in the late 1940s and was incorporated in 1951 as Al-Anon Family Groups, a primary source for wives, husbands, children, and significant others who live with or have their lives affected by an alcoholic. Today, Al-Anon is nationwide and international. It can be located through central offices in major cities throughout the United States. Members frequently describe Al-Anon as a place where people get their minds and hearts together. It is not group therapy, nor is it connected with a particular philosophy of explanation or treatment. The majority of its members are women. Historically, all of its early members were women who played a service and back-up function to early AA meetings. Today, the membership includes perhaps 20 percent males and 80 percent females.

As social roles evolve, change will be reflected in the membership of AA and Al-Anon. Note that while young people do attend Al-Anon meetings, they are as likely to attend Alateen meetings. Alateen is allied with Al-Anon and uses its literature and format. Both programs derive from AA's twelve-step format. Al-Anon meetings are not gripe sessions focusing on the behavior of the alcoholic. Instead, the meetings focus on methods, philosophy, and techniques that make living with the alcoholic better for those around him or her. Al-Anon is for people who, for a number of reasons, cannot flee. The approach is captured in the organization's three C's: (1) I did not *cause* the alcoholism; (2) I can't *control* it; and (3) I can't *cure* it. At meetings one hears: "The alcoholic hugs the bottle while the family hugs the drunk."

Al-Anon grew out of the difficulties that wives were experiencing in living with their alcoholic husbands early in the history of AA. Founded by Lois Wilson, Bill Wilson's wife, and a woman identified as Anne B., it is organizationally separate from AA, although it is not uncommon to find them sharing space or having Al-Anon meetings take place in one part of a building while AA meetings are going on in the other.[1]

As is the case with AA, Al-Anon meetings take place in homes, public buildings, churches, and similar locations. Like AA, they have a unique literature that is user specific. Although its charter is clear, it is frequently the gateway to AA. An individual may attend Al-Anon around issues of someone else's drinking and, in the stories and descriptions, come to find that their own drinking is problematic. As one AA member said, "I came to hear the music but I stayed to dance."

Al-Anon recognizes that while abstinence is a goal, the difficulties of the alcoholic do not end with the beginning of sobriety. It took the alcoholic a long while to act out his or her alcoholism, and it will take him or her a long while to learn how to behave nonalcoholically. The first year or two of sobriety can be characterized by irritability and self-absorption to the point of exclusion of others.

The significance of the effective nature of the Al-Anon group meeting cannot be over estimated. The functional dynamics of the group operate within a warm, sharing and emotionally supportive community. Despite differences in age, socioeconomic features and lifestyle, members have all experienced severe and often violent, fearful problems, common to house-holds and relationships where there is alcohol and abuse. This community constitutes a haven for those who felt their problems to be unique before they joined Al-Anon. It also allows them to observe successful role models who cope with problems they perceive to be more serious than their own. The homogeneity of the group in shared experiences provides a non-threatening arena that encourages comparison of coping strategies, intro-spection, and the possibilities of change. Members often point up the value of the membership being closed to alcoholics. In this supportive en-vironment, away from the alcoholic and the emotions his presence pro-vokes, the Al-Anon member can ventilate freely and develop a 'working the program.' Members are given telephone lists and urged to call other members at any hour of the day or night when they are in need of support. Some members have sponsors who introduce them to the group and coach them through early crises. But this is not a common pattern as in Alco-holics Anonymous. The culture of Al-Anon groups is remarkably stable from meeting to meeting. The most effective groups are those that have the most outspoken, long term members who embody, most articulately, the Al-Anon philosophy in their talks and their advice.[2]

Out of love, fear, or guilt, people closest to the alcoholic protect him or her from the consequences of their drinking. In doing so, they prevent the alco-holic from experiencing the devastating impact of alcohol on his or her life and prolong the final decision that must be made. Al-Anon works to inter-rupt that process. It is when the alcoholic is faced with consequences that he hopefully decides to do something about his alcoholism.

Wives stop being enablers when they focus on their own lives. They begin to see that they cannot change anyone, including their spouses. They refuse to help in ameliorating the circumstances of their spouses' drinking. Torn-up rooms are left unstraightened; spilled messes and vomit are left where they lie. Excuses are not made to anyone for any reason. Rather than being en-ablers, they live their lives for themselves. They don't argue about alcohol any more. Alcohol may run their spouses' lives, but it no longer runs theirs. They stop feeling sorry for themselves. They stop being victims.

Betty Z. at an Al-Anon meeting talked about awakening to the role she played in her husband's alcoholism. "Bill always drank, but it didn't become obvious to me that it was dominating his life until we had been married for fifteen years or so. We had three children. Bill worked on an airline job that necessitated his traveling, but he was always home on weekends. I began to notice that his hours were getting more and more erratic. It took quite a while, but it finally dawned on me that Bill had a drinking problem. The most obvious signs were long absences from home and an occasional dent in the car. His absences became more frequent, and his automobile accidents became more obvious.

"Finally, one night, coming back from a party, he got a DWI. I began talking to Bill about his drinking, asking him why he didn't slow down or why he couldn't just have a couple of drinks and leave it at that. I extracted promises from him about not getting drunk at parties that we attended. Bill assured me each time that he wouldn't, but each time, he did. It seemed that this was one area in our lives where he couldn't keep his word to me. I began finding bottles all over the house. Bill began stopping drinking, sometimes for a week, sometimes for two weeks, but it always seemed worse when he went back to it.

"Keep in mind that this was going on over a period of about five years. My anxieties and fears grew as Bill's problem with alcohol did. Trips to the liquor store were as frequent as trips to the supermarket, and it seemed that I was always restocking the refrigerator with beer and the bar with whiskey. It got to a point that I hated the sight of alcohol in any form. I wasn't a drinker myself. I just didn't like it. When Bill got drunk at parties, I called to apologize for him. I lied about him taking medication. I lied about his having the flu. I lied to friends in general. I was embarrassed for him. I was embarrassed by Bill's drunkenness. I was embarrassed for myself.

"In between periods of excessive drinking, Bill was the same sweet guy I had known through most of our years of marriage. He tried to be good and attentive to the kids and me, but it was difficult. He kept drinking through it all. Major events in the children's lives came and went; graduations, confirmations, proms, and so on. Bill was only vaguely aware of them, and at the few that he did attend, he managed to embarrass the entire family with his drinking. I started to feel I was living a soap opera.

"The kids had long since gotten to the point where they would prefer that their father not be around when they had friends over or when something was going on at school. It wasn't that they were hostile to their father; he was an embarrassment. We didn't know how much resentment the kids had about Bill's drinking. We were to find out about that later in family therapy. Each of the occasions of upset caused a major battle between Bill and me. I kept lying and making excuses for him and telling the kids that he was fundamentally okay and trying to hold our home together, but it was becoming increasingly difficult.

Bill seemed less and less concerned with us and more and more concerned with his drinking, which was now going on twenty-four hours a day. He refused to admit that he had a problem with alcohol and would storm out of the house in anger when I raised the subject. When he started wetting the bed at night, I started sleeping alone. That was the final straw. We weren't together anymore at all. I told Bill I was going to leave him many times, but I never did.

"After joining Al-Anon, I felt better about what was going on with me. I stopped lying for him, and I stopped making excuses for him. When he was too hung over to go to work and his boss called, I told the boss that Bill was too hung over to go to work. Bill was in a constant state of fury about my unwillingness to cooperate with him in maintaining deceptions about sobriety. I explained to the children that their father was an alcoholic and told them not to expect much from him. I tried to talk about the disease concept with them so that they would understand that their father was not volitionally being the embarrassment that he was. I stopped buying liquor of any kind and stopped getting Bill drinks when he wanted them.

"When he wanted to talk about his drinking, I refused. I told him I thought he was an alcoholic, was killing himself, and needed to do something about it. I suggested AA. Beyond that I did not argue. I did not point fingers of guilt; I simply ignored his drinking. If Bill came home at night and collapsed on the couch, I let him lay where he fell. I didn't put blankets on him. I didn't take his shoes off. I didn't try to make him comfortable. I just left him there in his own juices until he woke up. I was damned if I was going to help him drink anymore. I couldn't stop his drinking, but I didn't have to help him avoid the consequences of it.

"Unfortunately, it took a long time for Bill to wake up. He drank for several years after I joined Al-Anon. It was Al-Anon that helped me get through those years and helped me make sense of what was a painful and difficult situation. It helped me deal with the kids and their questions, and it in turn helped them understand what was going on in their lives. Bill blamed me for the loss of his job because when the boss called I was honest with him about Bill's drinking. I didn't make an issue of it and I didn't call to report on him, but I didn't lie when I was asked questions either.

"Bill finally wrecked the car and got a DWI. He was ordered to go to five AA meetings a week as a condition of his probation. Oh my, how he complained about that. 'Maybe he drank too much, but he wasn't that bad.' After Bill had been going to AA under the court supervision for seven or eight months, I got a call from his boss asking about Bill's condition. He remembered Bill as a good employee and regretted having to let him go. He couldn't continue anymore with Bill drinking all the time. We had a nice talk. I told him about Bill's AA involvement. He asked if I trusted it. I said I trusted it today. Bill eventually got his job back and has been sober for seven years. It still isn't easy between us, and I still have trouble trusting him. That's true for the kids also. But things are a lot better between us than they have been for years, and I am glad that my marriage held together."

Bill was lucky. He hit bottom and found AA. He was not a volunteer, but he went to meetings, got sober, and is sober today. His wife learned that Bill's sobriety is his own and not dependent on her in any way. In time she will learn to trust him again. It takes time. Chicanery and furtive behaviors characterize the alcoholic's relationship with his family in the later stages of his drinking. How could it be otherwise? He is obsessed with alcohol and cannot stop, while the momentum of the family is toward normalcy. The abuse of alcohol can only undermine the life processes that lead to family stability. Bill had to experience the consequences of his alcoholism. He had to make a connection between his drinking and what happened to him. This is extremely difficult to do because, as we've said before, alcoholism is a disease of denial.

The alcoholic's attitude toward his family can be an indicator of willingness to get sober as well as progress in early sobriety. Most alcoholics, when they first try to get sober, expect it to be business as usual with the exclusion of alcohol. They don't realize that many of their attitudes are going to need changing or that they are going to have to sort out the mess that is left behind. These things are necessary to sustain sobriety. Wally T. was talking about a man he sponsored a few years ago. He was careful not to identify the man in any way, arbitrarily calling him Lamar. Wally was talking about the need to deal with family matters and the necessity of defining alcoholism as a family disease.

"I met Lamar when I was called by a man I sponsored to go with him on a Twelve-Step call. A friend in AA, sober for eleven months, had gotten drunk. He was arrested in his home that night. His wife called the police when Lamar had loaded one of his guns and waved it around threatening to kill everyone at work. In the process of getting the gun, he had physically abused his wife. He had large stores of ammunition and guns all over the house because of his interest in target shooting and hunting. His wife bundled their five-year-old up, went to a neighbor's house, and called the police.

"It was lucky for Lamar that he was as meek as a lamb when the police arrived. He did not confront them with the gun but had laid it down before he answered the door. He was obviously drunk and creating a disturbance, so the police took him to the station and it was there that I went to see him. We introduced ourselves to the desk sergeant and asked if we could see Lamar. The desk sergeant wanted to talk about AA. He said he had an uncle who had been helped, and he thought it was a wonderful organization. I think it was for this reason that we were treated as well as we were. We were shown every courtesy.

"When we talked to Lamar, he had been there for about two hours and was getting aware enough to know what he had done. He was handcuffed to a radiator, sitting in a chair waiting for the wagon. He was withdrawn and full of remorse. He was worried about his wife and repeatedly asked why this was happening to him, what was going on. We simply said that this was happening to him because he was an alcoholic who drank. No other explanation seemed quite as direct and to the point.

"We managed to make an arrangement with the police for Lamar not to be charged but taken to the hospital for observation. He was taken to the alcohol unit of a local hospital that had a seven-day treatment program. This was not the first time that he had been hospitalized. The year before he had been hospitalized twice and gone through two twenty-eight-day programs. I went with his wife to see him in the hospital the next day. He seemed to be feeling better. He said that his drinking bout had lasted only two days and that it had been triggered by an ongoing upset at work. I didn't think this was the time to try to figure out the whys and wherefores of his drinking and said so. I wondered what his plans were, had he taken care of arrangements at work, and so on.

"As it turned out, his stay at the hospital lasted only two days. He resumed treatment contacts with the hospital where he had completed his last detox. He asked me to be his sponsor. I agreed, and over the next several months, I tried to work with him. Outside of the home, his wife was an assertive and pleasant woman who worked full time and was raising a daughter. In the home, she became a different person. When I visited, I would see her taking an obviously subservient role to Lamar. She jumped at his every command.

His daughter, on the other hand, was the focus of his solicitous attention, and he seemed to take delight in being manipulated by her. Lamar had been married before and had a son by that marriage. He had always supported his son. It was only later that I learned the extent to which Lamar used support and money to manipulate the boy.

"Our sponsorship relationship was bumpy from the start. At first I heard a lot from him, with requests for interpretation, advice, or just support. This disappeared as I began suggesting working the Steps to get at the reasons for his frequent slips. I suggested that he work the Steps and take a look at the extent to which his behavior had hurt other people.

"His wife called from time to time, talking about his indifference and describing Lamar as exactly the same person without the alcohol. She said she almost missed Lamar's passing out because it gave her some respite from his arrogance and his demands. She loved her husband but was frightened for him. She had seen this pattern repeated over and over. Even he was afraid he would drink. In a lot of ways, I agreed with her. Lamar resisted every attempt at change. Even after his last disastrous bout with drinking, he still wanted business as usual and sobriety on his terms. He was going to do exactly as he pleased, with no looking back and no interference. Throughout all of this he expressed a love and reverence for AA, its principles, and Steps. He just didn't do them.

"After about four months, I got a call from his wife. She was desperate. Lamar had gotten drunk and locked himself in their bedroom. He didn't have any guns with him, but there were guns all over the house again. She was scared to death. I advised her to gather up the guns and put them in a box, and told her that I would be right over.

"When I saw Lamar that night, he was still half full of booze and not making sense. It became clear why he could not get sober and stay sober. The impact his drinking was having on his family was also clear. Lamar ruled his house like a benevolent dictator. His wife had no idea how much money they had in the bank, how much he earned, or what became of the money she earned. In fact, she had nothing that she could call her own and had no idea of how finances were managed. Lamar maintained two accounts, one in both their names, with a minimal balance, and another in his name only. She had some idea of the insurance coverage but little else. I suggested that she begin attending Al-Anon meetings.

"That evening Lamar was threatening to leave her and the little girl. He said that he loved his wife but 'couldn't stand her.' He had mixed feelings about his life. It was clear that he didn't see alcohol as the root of any of his problems. He treated his alcoholism as if it were an attendant condition, something that he could take care of at his leisure while the rest of his life was ongoing. I left around two o'clock in the morning. Lamar went to bed.

"The next several weeks revolved around my attempts at getting Lamar to do a Fourth and Fifth Step and to begin assessing his behavior toward his family. I wanted him to see the relationship between how he behaved toward people and how they behaved toward him. He resisted every suggestion. I got fewer and fewer calls from him until finally I didn't hear from him at all. At meetings I asked him how he was doing and what was going on. The answer was always 'fine.' 'I am doing just fine.'

"In conversation with Lamar, I discovered that he was going to three, perhaps four meetings a week. Two of those meetings were therapy sessions run by the hospital and were not AA meetings. By my count, he was going to two AA meetings a week. I wasn't surprised that he was getting drunk. AA was his second choice in all things, and I didn't see that I could do any good by continuing as his sponsor. I had a talk with him and told him I thought he better find another sponsor because he and I weren't working out very well. He agreed.

"When last I heard, he was still trying to get another sponsor. I suspect that he was going to have a hard time finding one who would either leave him alone or give him the answers that he wanted. I am also certain that he is drinking again. I guess the point that I am making is that his attitude and his feelings toward his family—the manipulation, the selfishness, the need to control, the shallowness of relationships, and the single direction of things, all going his way—characterized his relationship with others in his immediate world."

The point of this story is, of course, that the person who stops drinking without addressing the alcoholism will drink again. A self-obsessed attitude and resistance to change does not produce sobriety or spiritual growth. Change has to be dictated by an analysis of past and current behaviors toward people. The driver of change is the ethical and moral foundations manifest in the Twelve Steps of AA. Individual changes are mandated by the need for sobriety and accomplished through working the Steps one at a time and in order. It is a sad fact that AA is not for everyone who needs it but for everyone who wants it. The lesson is simple. Half measures solve nothing. Those people who come into AA and work the Steps and the program enjoy change and stay sober; those who don't usually get drunk.

In Lamar's case, his attitudes toward his family mirrored his attitude toward the rest of the world. He wanted to stop drinking but he didn't want to inconvenience himself in any way or change. Consequently, he continued to drink. His wife enabled his drinking with her passivity and willingness to hop whenever he told her to. Her failure to insist on knowledge of the family finances or, for that matter, control over her own paycheck, enabled Lamar to continue playing the role of big shot and the dispenser of favors in the house. She was exactly where he wanted her, under his thumb. While she complained about his drinking, she never did anything to bring the consequences of his drinking home to him. She always forgave him and expressed hope for the future. She did this whether or not she believed that hope existed or really felt forgiveness.

Wally described Lamar's relationship to his five-year-old daughter. "He sure spent a lot of time buying things for that little girl. He was always telling stories about how cute she was and how old she was for her age. When I saw them interact, I saw him making a display of buying her affection and forcing his wife to play the role of disciplinarian. Although she corrected the child, there was obviously a warm loving relationship between them. The little girl seemed far more tentative around her father. When I visited Lamar the night of his arrest, I saw another side of his daughter. She cringed when she saw he was waking up and was crying when I entered the house. She looked at me with big, sad eyes and said, 'Daddy's drunk again and locked in the bedroom.' Her mother tried to shush her but she continued, 'help my daddy feel better.'

"He began promising her toys that he would buy for her tomorrow. He placed her in the middle of the bed and expected our conversation to go on around her. I asked him please to put the little girl to bed so that we could talk. He didn't see that we had much to talk about. I have always wondered why it is that children who are abused by their parents and are afraid of them seem to love the parents all the more for it. Lamar's alcoholism was destroying his family. His wife made faint stabs at a commitment to Al-Anon, but with working full time, raising her daughter, and running the house, her hours were pretty well filled. If he ever does get sober, this character has got a lot of amends to make."

Lamar's wife is an enabler. She is passive when she should confront, and she allows herself to be victimized by Lamar and his alcoholism. By being a doormat and opting for peace at any price, she aids Lamar in denying his alcoholism. Every time he gets drunk, then gets sober and picks up his life again, his feelings that everything is okay are reinforced. Lamar's wife needs to assume control of her own life and stop letting his alcoholism rule her. She needs to let Lamar bear the consequences for his drunkenness and to stop making excuses for him. She needs to demand her rights in the marriage and begin controlling her share of the family finances, and most certainly her own paycheck, to ensure her continued safety and that of her daughter. She needs to explain her husband's disease to her daughter and make it clear to her that she is not responsible for what is happening to him. The child is the one in the family who is in need of explanation and protection. Lamar's wife needs to assert herself and, most importantly, find time in her life for Al-Anon.

The alcoholic's perception of his family and the impact of his alcoholism on family members are almost always skewed. He frequently defines his role in the family in terms of services. "I supported them. I always worked. They never wanted for anything. The only person I hurt is myself." When the alcoholic gains in sobriety, his attitude toward the family changes. Likewise, he is forced to examine what he has done to his family. He can make amends. I have heard countless alcoholics describe discharging a portion of their amends by living a sober purposeful life that includes loving concern for the family. Some things simply require forgiveness. Some fences are never mended. The point is that it takes time for the alcoholic to gain perspective on the family. It takes time to gain focus and balance.

Edward B. is a tall, thin man. He speaks with a deep, slow drawl unimpeded by teeth. He has been sober for a long time and is known for driving bunches of newly sober people around to meetings in a van bought for that purpose. People like to hear him because he has a sense of humor about what has happened to him.

"You know, when I was drinking, I spent all my time at the bar down the street. If I needed anything, that's were I went to shop. I bought everything the bar sold: combs, toenail clippers, snacks, pickled eggs. If they didn't have it, I didn't need it. The bar was my entire focus. Everyone I knew was there. I saw them in waves. Groups came and went all day. I was there to greet them all. I spent time at home when I didn't have any money. My wife worked, the kids worked, and I pretended to look for work. I drove a cab, did odd jobs and whatever pick-up work I could find. I lied about how much I earned so I could drink. I was really nuts. I would walk all the way downtown to sell blood for $7.50 a pint, and I would walk all the way back to save carfare. As soon as I would get to the bar, I heard myself ordering drinks for everyone. But I never gave anything at home.

"Through all of this, my wife was loyal to me. She didn't put me out. My kids wanted nothing to do with me. My wife paid for just about everything. This went on for years. When I went to AA and got sober, she didn't trust it. The kids didn't want to hear about it. I got a job driving a truck and started bringing money home. Boy, did I think I was something. I expected to be praised to the heavens for doing what regular people do every day of their lives. After about three years had gone by, I started to feel that my wife wasn't good enough for me. I worked all day and went to AA every night. I hauled people around, and they told me how wonderful I was. I forgot that I had been a bum for thirty years.

"I'm grateful now that my wife stayed with me. We do all right, but I remember when I told her I was tired of her the way she was. She said that she was tired too. She called me a no-good bum and asked how much I thought I had changed. She really gave me hell. She let me know just what I was like. I heard a lot of things I didn't want to hear. She said that if there was any good in me she was going to stick around to get the benefit of it. She had had all the rest. I started working the Steps after that. I'm trying to make it up to my family every day."

Attitudes are frequently slow to change; years of drinking leave residuals that take time to recognize and even more time to change. Attitudes toward the family require scrutiny.

Parents with Children Who Abuse Alcohol

As many parents say, having children is a blessing. And, while it doesn't seem fair, those cute little bundles grow into people. As children grow older and enter school, friends and peer groups become the primary source of socialization. Parental influence diminishes. Unfortunately, parental responsibilities and plans for their children do not diminish. What parents want for children frequently conflicts with what children want for themselves. While age is no guarantor of wisdom, youth appears to mitigate against it. Most parents in the last three decades have had to contend with youthful rebellion, the recreational use of dangerous drugs, and a culture that panders to youth in almost every way. It's a tough time to raise kids. In the late 1970s and early 1980s, a lot of parents breathed a sigh of relief when the youthful allegiance to getting high switched from drugs to booze. Feelings of relief were premature. As reported in the popular press, it is now generally agreed that alcohol abuse is the single most serious health problem among young people today.

When drugs were the vogue, some kids seemed to be able to experiment with and even use certain nonnarcotic drugs over a period of time and then stop with no apparent long-range effects. Some tried them and were not that interested. Others tried them and were caught up in increasing drug dependence, use, and a degenerating lifestyle. Most parents found themselves powerless in the face of this combination of forces.

Hugh O. was talking about the nature of addictions and vulnerability at an Al-Anon meeting. The subject of drugs had come up, and he compared the situations that the parents of drug abusers face with the problems faced by parents of teenage alcoholics. "I have known Larry since he was three years old. He has always called me 'uncle,' and although the title is honorary, the relationship has always been real. His brother and sister, one older and one younger, grew up in the same home and in the same neighborhood and with much the same kinds of friends without any difficulties with substance abuse. Larry somehow got involved with drugs. He drank, but drugs were his choice.

"At first, no one noticed. When his parents realized he was coming home stoned, they began the usual round of control efforts: forbidding him to see his friends or go out, visiting school counselors, and so on. Larry continued to do what he wanted to do. His use of hallucinogens took over his life. He painted his room black with little gold stars on the ceiling and began to talk in religious parables. He would disappear for days at a time, sometimes weeks. It was discovered that he was going up into Canada to visit friends who lived unsupervised. They had the run of a large home in a rural area, and all of them were into drugs and sexual experimentation.

"The more his parents tried to control him, the more uncontrollable he got. He was a big kid and got violent around the house a few times, smashing up his own guitars and furniture and threatening his parents. The police were unable to do anything for the family unless they were willing to press charges for assault, which they were not willing to do. Larry never seemed to have any drugs in his possession. No one really knew what he was taking, and he didn't talk about it. At a much later time, we all learned that Larry's drug of choice

was PCP. He was dismissed from school in his senior year after climbing the
school flagpole and talking to the school counselor about voices telling him to
do things. He was convinced that he could fly and that he was the reincarnation of the Son of God. He began to take on the clinical aspects of schizophrenia, and the school felt that they could no longer deal with him.

"Because he was sixteen years old at the time, his parents were still responsible for him and were ordered by the juvenile court to keep him at home and
supervise him carefully. He had been brought before the court on a burglary
charge. He and a friend had broken into another friend's house in search of
prescription drugs. They had found some tranquilizers, taken them, and
fallen asleep on the floor, where they were discovered the next morning by the
returning parents. They were arrested.

"By this time, Larry was hallucinating on a regular basis, was still taking
drugs whenever he could get them, and was uncontrollable at home. When in-
terfered with seriously, he simply disappeared. His parents were in a quandary.
They finally talked Larry into seeing a psychiatrist, who diagnosed him as
having schizophrenia and put him on a combination of drugs geared to alleviate his symptoms. He gained weight, shook a lot, and withdrew within himself. He needed treatment. Rather then send him to a public institution, his
parents spent their life savings and mortgaged their home to send him to a
private school dealing with children with drug and psychiatric problems. By
this time it was impossible to separate Larry's personality from the damage
that had been done to his brain from smoking PCP.

"Larry is now twenty-two years old. He had been brain damaged by his use
of PCP and is educationally and emotionally about seventeen years of age. He
is not suited for work of any type after spending four years in a residential
treatment program. In that period of time, he was not able to finish his high
school diploma. His parents, however, grew during that four-year period.
They remain hopelessly in debt and will be paying off school bills until they
are in their seventies. Larry's treatment costs were well beyond what they
could afford.

"During his period of residence at the school, however, his parents learned
to separate his problems from their own. When he left the school for the last
time, he was told not to come home. They still talk to him and wish him well
and hope that he can manage. They have, however, separated his problems
from their own. He will have to deal with the consequences of his behavior.
Larry seems to be taking positive steps toward accepting responsibility for his

life. He has been receiving limited financial assistance from the state and is in a sheltered workshop trying to learn how to support himself."

All the lives in the family were affected by Larry's drug abuse. The effect will continue as long as his parents have serious debts resulting from Larry's treatment. It took years for them to understand that they had done everything that they could do and that it was necessary for them to find peace in their own lives. This particular story did not have a happy ending. When last heard from, Larry was drinking heavily. He seemed to think that drinking was all right as long as he stayed away from street drugs. Those in AA know only too well the close connection between any mood-altering substances and alcohol.

Some kids seem to be more vulnerable to alcohol and drugs than others. Some parents enable their children and hope that they will come out of it and go on to live normal lives. Some do; some don't. Some parents practice what has come to be known as "tough love," cutting their children off—no money, no car, no support—until they are clean of drugs. Some stay marginal. What parents do or do not do appears to be irrelevant to the track of alcohol and drugs in the lives of their children. Those who handle the crisis most effectively separate their lives from the problems of their children. They separate what they can control from what they cannot control and learn to live with the latter.

When vulnerability makes itself known in children, whether it is to drugs, alcohol, or both, the children themselves are the custodians of their condition. They alone can effect a cure. Parents can aid in this process. They can refuse to be enablers. They can contribute, but they cannot control. They can teach but should not entreat. They must bring adult judgment to the process of change. They cannot allow the problems or addiction of their children to direct, circumscribe, or ruin their lives. Eventually, they must allow their children to suffer the consequences of their own behavior and their decisions about using.

In the past ten years, an increasing number of teenagers and people in their early twenties have joined AA. Many of these people describe themselves as having dual addictions. They put alcohol first and drugs second. The connection between the two is inescapable. The switch from drugs to alcohol all too frequently results in alcoholic dependence. It is not clear how vulnerability to one mood-altering substance is related to the other, but the implications for parents are the same. If parents wish to avoid being enablers, they must be aware of the symptoms of abuse and establish rules about how children use the house and family resources. Parental roles with underage children are complicated by a network of legal and moral obligations. It may be necessary to provide a roof and basic support despite a child's continued substance abuse.

Perhaps the hardest thing for parents to give up is the idea that they control their children. They can set examples, influence, and suggest, but they cannot control. It's a difficult tightrope to walk. Their role becomes better defined when they recognize that alcoholism and drug abuse are family problems. When the child in question is ready to end the abuse, he or she will look for solutions. The solutions may well be sought at home, provided home has not become a battleground. When alcoholism occurs in teens or preteens a bottom may occur early in family life. A defined problem may generate a solution. Fortunately, kids heal quickly. Physical recovery, unfortunately, frequently promises controlled drinking in the future. Alcoholism is a disease of denial. The course of alcoholism is always the same regardless of the age of onset. Alcohol does not know how old or how young you are.

Alcoholic kids are frequently in trouble. Kids in trouble inspire guilt in their parents. They also provoke anger, terror, frustration, hopelessness, and a myriad of other negative emotions that affect the family. They lie, cheat, steal, and defy any control that gets between them and alcohol. Families must learn to live one day at a time, to control what they can control, and to accommodate to the rest. Couples must cooperate absolutely to provide the best situation for the child involved. When parents don't cooperate, the child is at even greater risk of being lost. When a child turns eighteen, separate living arrangements may be necessary, but until that time, provisions for care must be made. Residential treatment facilities or high-security schools are available to families. They are, however, expensive and not viable options for everyone. As for the problem-defined schools, many professionals question their effectiveness. In most cases, they only seem to postpone the inevitable. Public facilities, unfortunately, often involve police authorities. Criminal incarceration at any level is invariably pernicious. It is curious that there appear to be more drug programs in the public domain than there are programs aimed at alcoholism among the young. For the young alcoholic, AA is still the best means of getting and staying sober. Involving the courts and public agencies often does more harm than good.

Parents Who Drink

One would think that growing up with the examples of drunken parents or parents who are sober in Alcoholics Anonymous would warn children of their own vulnerability and make alcohol less appealing. For many, this is not the case. Children of alcoholic parents are at risk for alcoholism. It is not at all unusual for them to have brothers, sisters, and cousins in AA. Alcoholics investigating their family trees almost invariably find alcoholics liberally distributed among the branches.

Scully T. is a big Swede from Minnesota. He has worked as a lumberjack and in oil rigs in the Southwest. He cuts quite a colorful figure and has been sober in AA for many years. He describes his initial surprise at coming up alcoholic.

"After my first few meetings at AA, I began to get an inkling of what was wrong with me. I wasn't just bound for trouble all my life. I wasn't just crazy. I was relieved to find out that I was an alcoholic. More importantly, I was relieved to find out that I could do something about my alcoholism and start to turn my life around. I was thirty-three years old when I got to AA, and in those thirty-three years I had been arrested many times for assault and battery. I had a history of drinking my money away. I made good money, but I had nothing to show for it. I had never gotten married because I never stayed in one place long enough to establish a relationship with a woman. I had few friends because of all of my moving around. Every job I ever had was one where drinking was expected. Those were the kinds of jobs I gravitated to.

"I came to AA because I didn't want to live the way I was living anymore and couldn't seem to stop it. I seemed to be drunk all the time. In fact, it was a woman who got me to AA. She stayed sober for a few months and then got drunk. I stayed sober. Anyway, the point that I'm making is that after I started feeling better, I wondered why I became alcoholic. I kept hearing about family histories of alcoholism, but I couldn't remember anyone in my family having a drinking problem. I talked to my parents about it, and little by little an interesting picture emerged.

"They began denying that anybody in the family had a drinking problem and then began to talk about certain family members who drank quite a bit. Before you know it they were describing relatives in Sweden on my mother's side who had died young after mysterious circumstances or who had the reputation of having drunk themselves to death. Alcoholics came out of the woodwork. My father described his own father as a man who would go to bed for weeks on end drinking, not even stirring himself to go to the bathroom. He used a chamber pot. His wife put up with all of this because the old man terrorized the family. I had never heard my father describe his father in anything other than hateful terms. The more I heard, the more I was convinced that my grandfather was alcoholic.

"One of the most curious stories my father told me was about a half-brother that was sixteen years older than he was. Dad had never thought of him as an alcoholic; he just thought of him as crazy. One Thanksgiving Day, this brother, Sven, got up from the dinner table and excused himself, saying he was going to the washroom. He walked out the front door and was never seen again. Dad laughed at this. He said that no one knew what happened to Sven. Wherever he went, he was down the drain as far as the family was concerned."

Sven's parents were not alcoholic, neither of them drank. For some reason, alcoholism frequently skips a generation. I remain convinced, however, of the heredity link. Throughout the country, AA chapters are being founded specifically for the sons and daughters of alcoholic parents. It is obvious that the example set by alcoholic parents cannot counteract the influence of a biological vulnerability once alcohol is introduced to the system.

For the alcoholic, a family is frequently a source of guilt. They are recipients of the amends alcoholics make as they work the Steps toward sobriety. Alcoholics must get sober for themselves. Before they can learn to forgive others and to accept forgiveness from others, they must learn to forgive themselves. Before they can learn to love someone else selflessly, they must learn to love themselves. This is a difficult and daunting task. There is an old saying in AA that when you are not good for anything else and not good for yourself, you are just right for AA.

Scully did not experience the alcoholism of his extended family, and he became alcoholic despite the nonalcoholic environment of his nuclear family. His family had not warned him about his possible vulnerability to alcoholism. He, therefore, did not understand the progression of his drinking. Children who grow up in an alcoholic family are vulnerable on two fronts. They may have a genetic predisposition to alcoholism and must cope with the influence of a chaotic alcoholic home.

We Learn to Dance at Home

Our families of origin are our primary source of socialization until individuation begins and we are influenced by peer groups and other social institutions. The family is the support system, emotional and physical, throughout childhood, adolescence, and early adulthood. Needless to say, families are variously equipped to perform these all-important tasks. In addition to providing a genetic heritage, families provide social and intellectual frameworks within which individuals can work out the various potentials of their being. In this sense, families provide horizons and limit the possible range of behaviors in every social interaction. Families are frequently the origins of an individual's sense of self. Families begin or hinder the development of a child's sense of fit in the world. Families teach by word, and, more importantly, they teach by example.

The rights and wrongs, the "normal" and "abnormal" of alcohol use are taught by example in families. Family structure and social status can foster or discourage what exists as biological potential in any child. I recall a patient talking about his early childhood and his initial university experiences. He talked about the fact that as much as he wanted to drink through high school, he was unable to because he had no money. The money that he earned went to his family and went to his own support. His time was likewise restricted because he went to school full time and worked twenty-five hours per week. This left little time for partying. He did note that he drank enthusiastically when he had the chance. He thought this was normal.

The same was true of his university experience. He worked at two jobs, night and day, in order to pay tuition, room, and board. Between a heavy university schedule and a heavy work schedule, he had little time to drink or to attend parties where drinking was the norm. When he had the opportunity, he drank and was enamored of drinking but was unable to do anything about it. He assumed all of his feelings about alcohol were perfectly normal. He thought a lot about liquor, thought about buying it when he could, and when he did buy some, he drank it all immediately. He assumed all of these behaviors were normal. He came from a family that did not drink. He did not experience the casual use of alcohol. His role models were his peers who were profligate in their use of alcohol. It came out later that his father had had considerable difficulty with alcohol when he was a young man. When he had married, his new wife had insisted that he "take the pledge." The father had not had a drink since. The young man's mother never drank. They did not enjoy a large, extended family, and so my patient's range of experience was very small. When he found himself with time on his hands and money in his pocket, he began to drink in a pathological way. Within ten years he was treated for alcoholism at a local hospital.

There are many types of families, all of which are charged with the same tasks of socialization for their children. They include many variations in structure. There are single-parent families, traditional two-parent families, and blended families with parents holding multiple allegiances and unrelated children living together. There are families with firm structure and expectations and families who do not plan beyond the day. Regardless of structure, all families provide the social and behavioral horizons of their children, or at least the beginnings of these orientations.

In any event, children are better off being informed of alcoholic patterns existing in their families. They should be told what these patterns mean and how to prepare for the eventuality of their own possible alcoholism.

8

THE ROAD TO A LIFE WELL LIVED

THE PROMISES

The meeting on Pine Street begins promptly at 8:30 p.m. It takes place in a small auxiliary building behind a church referred to in the community as "The Cathedral." The large meeting room is warm, and a breeze goes through it, encouraged by a large fan in the doorway. The walls are covered with pictures drawn or painted by children who use the room during the day as part of a preschool program sponsored by the women of the church. In its use as an AA meeting room, the tables are put together in a circle, with a head table in front of the large stage that dominates the end of room.

There has been the usual clatter of coffee making and cookie distribution. The Prologue has been read, and the Steps and Traditions have been read, as well as a bulletin sent by Intergroup citing meetings or activities of particular interest. The meeting's speaker stands at the head table and begins. She is a tall, imposing, well-groomed, angular woman. Her voice has a cadence, and her language is so precise that her background in teaching is immediately evident.

"My name is Edwina, my friends call me Eddie. I come from hardscrabble farming people on the Eastern Shore. My parents were . . . I guess if they were down South, you'd call them sharecroppers. On the Shore, they were tenants, farming a section of land that was part of a larger landholding of a horse farm. My father raised soybeans and corn. My mother raised children and tried to keep the boat of our family on top of the water rather than under it. My brothers—I had four of them—helped Dad work the farm from the moment they could hold an implement. All left home in their middle to late teens after a fragmented education and years of hard work. They seemed to know that whatever the future held for them, it was not in farming or in the little community that was our world.

"I was the youngest of the children and, as clearly as I can recall, was final witness to my mother's frustrations and my father's exhaustion. While I was in school, I came to the attention of one of the nuns who taught English and poetry. Under the starch and rustle of her habit, she was a warm, kind person. When it came time for me to leave school to join the economic struggles of my family, she intervened with my mother and offered an opportunity for me to continue my education at a boarding school. The school was a stepping-stone to university training and also to the religious life. My mother let me go.

"I began entry into an intellectual life that opened the beauty of the world to me and a religious life that restricted my participation in it. I lived and worked as a teaching nun in the inner city. I lived in a large house with a number of other nuns. Some wore habits; some didn't. We taught at St. Arlis in the neighborhood. No one knew quite who St. Arlis was, and among ourselves we referred to him as the patron saint of agony and sore feet. In many ways, I began to feel as lost as St. Arlis himself.

"My drinking began with an occasional beer or cocktail at neighborhood functions. It quickly escalated into alcohol being a source of energy and comfort to me. I began drinking before I went to bed in order to sleep comfortably. My escalation into dependence and alcoholism was a seamless rocket ride. My drinking was both open and secretive at this time in my career, and I rapidly progressed into hiding my drinking and the amount that I drank from everyone. I called passing out in the afternoon taking a power nap. Little by little, my peculiar behavior became the subject of talk in the school and in the neighborhood. Finally, I was called to task by the Mother Superior of my order.

"While a nun, I was never able to get a handle on my drinking. The last several years of my religious career were punctuated by periods of frustrated abstinence and periods of drunkenness. After a final drying out in upper New York State, I came clean with members of my order about my addiction to alcohol and my conviction that whatever my spiritual or emotional need, I would not find resolution in the religious life.

"I came to realize it was not a life I had chosen but rather one that had been chosen for me. I became a teacher in the public school system and began to drink again. After about three years of continued drinking, I fell down in the classroom and hit my head on one of the desks, sustaining a concussion and a large cut. I was taken to a hospital, where I was visited by a priest. He was not visiting in his priestly capacity. He himself was an alcoholic and thought that he could relate to my experiences and, with luck, hook me up with AA. He took me to my first seven or eight meetings.

"At the meetings I found what I had not found in other aspects of my life. I found a spiritual sense of belonging that I had not experienced elsewhere. I found that doing the Steps provided a framework with which I could mechanically go about putting a floor under my everyday activities. Those no longer included drinking alcohol.

"The Promises have come true for me. They are manifest in the everyday aspects of my life. I am able to face the future with a sense of humor rather than a sense of dread. The spiritual aspect of my program grew as my experience in AA grew and as I was able to make the program my yardstick of behavior. I think my sense of spirituality grew out of the feeling of belonging and interaction with other alcoholics. I have come to believe that interaction with our fellow beings is the foundation of all spirituality in our lives. My religious beliefs have little to do with the spirituality I have derived from my ongoing involvement with AA. I hope you like me. I intend to spend my life here."

Spirituality and Sobriety

After the meeting, Eddie was asked if other members of her family were alcoholic and if she stayed in touch with her brothers. Eddie said that on reflection it was clear that her father had a problem with alcohol. He drank whenever he could. Poverty was his primary control. Her mother didn't drink at all. Two of her brothers were in the program out in California. She had less contact with her other brothers. Eddie's story makes one thing clear. The evolution of spirit occurs concomitantly with the ongoing practice of sobriety.

Eddie's life reflects the manifestation of the Promises. Her life is, in many ways, a construct of the Steps, the philosophy, and the fellowship of Alcoholics Anonymous. The crafting of Eddie's life required her dedication and the willingness to change along spiritual lines. Her spiritual condition is ensured by her continued involvement with AA and the practice of Steps Ten, Eleven, and Twelve, sometimes called the maintenance Steps. We all change.

Change is inevitable. The direction of that inevitability is our task. Spiritual evolution is a byproduct of a life well lived.

If you have read this far, you know all of the secrets. If you are reading to understand more about the alcoholic and how he or she feels about his or her alcoholism, you should have more insight into the subject. If you read this book because you think you may have a problem with alcohol yourself and want to know what to do about it, you have become aware of the most successful program in dealing with alcoholism today. Eddie's story reflects most of the salient points I have made so far about alcoholics.

Alcoholics are many and varied and yet share certain commonalities. They share a vulnerability to alcohol addiction. They share other personality characteristics produced by alcohol abuse. Eddie is not a "reformed" person. She is not a bad person made good. She is making different decisions in her life. Neither alcoholism nor its treatment has anything to do with moral issues or issues of willpower. Alcoholics are not weak people unable to control themselves any more than allergic persons are weak because they cannot control their allergies. Their moral and social choices are compromised by alcohol. They face great difficulty in getting sober in a culture that mandates drinking alcohol on almost every social occasion, defining it as a stepping-stone to maturity and independence.

I have described and had alcoholics describe, in their own words, the pernicious effect of alcohol on the body and life of the alcoholic. Because the topic has been recovery, I have drawn my examples from recovering alcoholics. I have emphasized success rather than failure. Obviously, there are failures in any program of recovery. Contrary to common interpretation, I view these as failures of the individual rather than failures of the program. "Seldom have we seen a person fail who has followed our path." When Bill Wilson was asked what he would change in the Big Book if he could, he said he would change *seldom* to *never*.

The Compulsion to Drink

Practicing alcoholics have little or no insight into their compulsion to drink. In general, they feel that they drink because they want to or because alcohol is the glue that holds them together and helps them cope with a hostile world. Recovery interrupts that process of alcoholic drinking and begins the process

of restoring the body to some kind of biochemical balance. After this inter-
ruption has occurred and treatment is ongoing, the period of reconstruction
can begin. During this period, the mental and the spiritual aspects of the disease are treated.

Unfortunately, the physical aspect of the disease is most clearly defined
symptomatically and is the most immediately amenable to treatment. This
results in increased vulnerability during this early period of abstinence. Physical recovery convinces the alcoholic that he or she is not alcoholic after all
and that the whole thing was a mistake. The cycle of dependence remains un-
broken, and the individual will drink alcoholically again before the other two
aspects of this disease are treated effectively. Any approach to the treatment
of alcoholism must include approaches to all three aspects (spiritual, physical, and mental) of the disease. Anything else is doing only part of the job.

Regardless of whether or not early drinking brings relief from psychological stress, alcoholics do not drink because they have problems. To the contrary, they have problems because they drink. Alcoholics do not abuse alcohol
for any reason other than that they are alcoholic. The addiction or compulsion to drink circumscribes their range of choices of behaviors or solutions.
The addiction attaches to all circumstances, regardless of potential outcomes.
The disease manifests itself in the life of drinkers at various times. Some are
instant alcoholics. They get into trouble when they drink and drink exces-
sively from the first time they drink. With others, the vulnerability is less and
manifests itself later in life.

Alcoholics do not drink because they are creative, highly complex, deeply
troubled, irresponsible, or anything else. For the alcoholic there are hundreds
of excuses for drinking, none of which address the compulsive nature of the
drinking. There are no relevant explanations that deal with the real reason
they drink. Stopping or slowing down is always a future possibility but a present impossibility. The alcoholic is not truly frightened of anything except giving up alcohol. Symptoms of all kinds are accommodated; the alcoholic stops
drinking when the price of admission is so high that he can no longer pay it.

I have heard it said, critically, that people in AA seem to have transferred
their dependence and obsession from alcohol to AA. All in all, I think, not a
bad transfer. In any given population of AA members, there will be those
whose lives seem to revolve around AA meetings, AA members, and AA activities, and others for whom the meetings and the interactions are less the focal
point in their lives. A strong tradition of service exists in AA. It is a part of the

Steps (particularly 10, 11, and 12) and a mandate in the practice and literature of the program. Attendance at meetings is a form of service. It shows the new-comer that long-term sobriety is a reality. How often has it been said, "When I first came to AA I was astounded that there were people who went three months without drinking"? If we think of AA activities and meetings as a ser-vice of affirmations, their role in ongoing sobriety becomes clear. You will never hear a sober person in the program wanting to return to the drunken life. In fact, a nostalgic description of drinking experiences is a sign of poten-tial trouble. No one denies that at one time alcohol "worked." The focus is on how alcohol stopped working and the unintended consequences of its use.

An individual member's involvement with and time spent in AA activities may vary throughout his or her sober career. Does this constitute depend-ence? I leave the answer to you. Some people who define themselves as alco-holic and seek help outside of Alcoholics Anonymous in one type of therapy or another do stop drinking, at least for a time. The overwhelming majority of these alternative approaches are less than effective, and studies indicate that without some type of ongoing support and means of normalization, al-coholics return to drinking. A life free of alcohol must be based on an aware-ness of biological vulnerability and the need for a particular life regime. For some reason, it is easier to understand and accept a life regimen that requires medication to alleviate symptoms than it is to understand a disease that re-quires changes in priorities and lifestyle.

There are also those who attend Alcoholics Anonymous meetings for vary-ing periods, usually a year or two, and then simply fall away from the program. It seems that the longer one is sober in the program, the better chance of re-maining sober the rest of one's life. The breaking point appears to be five years. After five years of sobriety, of those who remain in the program, about 95 per-cent stay sober. It is difficult to give statistics on people who leave the program after two or even three years of active participation because no one keeps track of them. For those who stay sober after leaving the program, it is clear that their lives have been altered permanently. The successful ones that I have talked with have incorporated the ethical and moral foundations of the AA program into their lives and are living it. They may attend meetings occasion-ally but not often. Perhaps they were the less afflicted. There are no satisfactory answers to these questions. Those who leave the program and get drunk obvi-ously didn't believe that it was the first drink that got them drunk. Perhaps they came to believe they were not alcoholic. Perhaps they simply succumbed to that body of rationalizations that every alcoholic is familiar with defining him or her as normal and capable of "handling the situation this time, because I know so much more about it." "This time it will be different."

Alcoholics who wonder whether they can leave the program and live the sober life must ask: What is the nature of the bet being made? What is at risk? In fact, life is at risk. Once an alcoholic drinks again, there is no guarantee that he or she will experience another recovery. It is sad but true that those who continually experiment with alcohol after they have discovered their own alcoholism seldom attain sobriety. The majority seem to live from one drunken episode to the next with varying periods of sobriety in between. No alcoholic seeking help has to settle for this kind of outcome. For those who work the Steps, there are the Promises. Our speaker Eddie managed to live them.

I cited the Promises in the discussion of the Steps in chapter 5. They are cited here again for clarity. The connection between achieving a sense of spiritual awareness and attaining the Promises in AA is clear. It is no accident that the Promises appear in the Big Book after a discussion of the first nine Steps. You will recall that the last three Steps of the twelve-step program were designated as the synoptic Steps, or the maintenance Steps. They are maintenance Steps because they serve to ensure that one is daily practicing each of the nine preceding Steps in their most complete sense.

The Promises

If we are painstaking about this phase of our development, we will be amazed before we are half way through. We are going to know a new freedom and a new happiness. We will not regret the past nor wish to shut the door on it. We will comprehend the word serenity and we will know peace. No matter how far down the scale we have gone, we will see how our experience can benefit others. That feeling of uselessness and self-pity will disappear. We will lose interest in selfish things and gain interest in our fellows. Self-seeking will slip away. Our whole attitude and outlook upon life will change. Fear of people and of economic insecurity will leave us. We will intuitively know how to handle situations which used to baffle us. We will suddenly realize that God is doing for us what we could not do for ourselves.

Are these extravagant promises? We think not. They are being fulfilled among us—sometimes quickly, sometimes slowly. They will always materialize if we work for them.[1]

What does each of these promises have to do with sobriety or spirituality? Virtually all of the Promises address the attainment of the spiritual life. As the Big Book says, "The spiritual life is not a theory. *We have to live it.*"[2] A life based on principles that lead to spiritual awareness or peace is sometimes difficult to find in this culture. Spirituality is not that evident in our interaction with the environment, whereas some cultures manage the integration nicely. Certain Native American tribes (the Hopi, notably) live according to their spiritual conception of the world daily. Their vision of the spirituality of man provides the moral and ethical benchmarks for all behavior. This ideal is the ultimate goal of the AA program. It is all-inclusive, and in its completeness it impels one toward the spiritual life.

The spiritual life of Western culture is not uniformly defined anywhere. Each culture defines its ideals of spirit differently. This definition of spirit is but a facet of the cultural meaning that defines spiritual road signs—that is, the guideposts of life lived to good purpose. That these spiritual life meanings are derived of interaction is evident in their being commonly held or revered among people. We are all aware of the stirring of this spirituality. Some call it an instinct of right or correctness. Some call it conscience while others have called it revelation. Regardless of its designation, in a world of evolving "morals" and "styles of behavior," certain constants of behavior and commonly held regulations of the rightness and wrongness of things have pertained, commonly understood throughout history. They are the stuff of AA.

When the alcoholic comes to AA, he or she is seldom a volunteer. Physical symptoms; chaotic lives; loss of loved ones, jobs, and property; the court; or physical collapse bring the lucky ones to AA. Some come directly. Some become involved in the program through hospitals, detox centers, or private physicians. Regardless of how they are introduced to the program, their success in sobriety and their longevity in the program depend on their involvement with the Steps. There is no way around it. The healing of the threefold nature of the disease of alcoholism requires a specific approach and life regimen. It is nice that a byproduct of the life regime is happiness, a sense of fit in the world of people and meaning and a deep perception of the spiritual life.

In earlier chapters I discussed the Steps, their intention, their impact, and how they work in the life of the alcoholic. I considered both the secular interpretations of the Steps and the more religiously (defined in the most neutral way) oriented interpretations. The Steps, in their inclusion in life, become more in "sum total" than they are separately. They gain strength in combination. Each Step is a part of a progression leading eventually to greater spiritual awareness. The spiritual awareness we relate to is not a contemplative, ethereal kind of awareness. It is, rather, spirituality reflected in interaction with one's fellows based on honesty, kindness, and a sense of empathy. One has a sense of having made peace with one's self and of an appropriate fit in the culture. The basic existential questions are answered. There is an acceptance of life on life's terms. It is a feeling of hope and faith in a life process that guarantees that things will be fundamentally all right. The way they ought to be. Not necessarily the way we want them to be, but the way they ought to be. This is a common theme in AA meetings.

That is what the Promises are all about. They are the logical results of the alcoholic's dealing with the past and its consequences, coming to grips with the disease and its implications of vulnerability, and owning change in the existential definitions that compromise his or her world of meaning. The AA literature says that the Promises are "being fulfilled among us—sometimes quickly, sometimes slowly. They will always materialize if we work for them." There are those in AA who say that you can spot the people for whom the Promises have materialized, even in part. They are the winners. They become the old-timers in AA. Newcomers are advised to stick with them. These are the people who come to mind when people in the program use the well-worn phrase to a newcomer: "If you want what we have and are willing to go to any length to achieve it . . ."

The "any length" they refer to, of course, is the application of the Steps in one's life. What they expect the newcomer to want is reflected in the eyes and in the very presence of those who have worked the Steps and begun to see the Promises working in their lives. This is why, in many ways, old-timers in AA identify the word *serenity* with the word *sobriety*. Anything less than serenity is simply the absence of alcohol or not being drunk. As we have said before, for alcoholics, half measures simply will not work. On their own, they may be able to stay dry for long periods of time or perhaps even forever, but they will never be fulfilled in life or approach an understanding of the threefold nature of their disease. Indeed, the spiritual life is not a theory. It must be lived.

"If we are painstaking about this phase of our development, we will be amazed before we are half way through." Consideration of the Promises, therefore, begins with the assumption that the alcoholic has carefully, thoroughly, and honestly completed the first nine Steps of the program. He has admitted that his life was unmanageable. He knows that he is powerless over alcohol and has accepted that he cannot get sober alone but requires a source of power outside himself. Additionally, he has recognized that to continue drinking in the face of the physical, psychological, and social costs is insanity. He has made a searching and fearless moral inventory, meaning a written list of weaknesses and personality characteristics, either directly or indirectly related to drinking. He has discussed this list with another individual with explicit willingness to have these defects of character corrected and is ready to accept help in this process. He has organized an itinerary of amends based on individuals who have been harmed either directly or indirectly by his drinking.

Throughout this process the alcoholic has come to rely on and has become involved in the daily regimen and program of Alcoholics Anonymous, including service to other alcoholics and daily (or more frequent) attendance at AA meetings. He has agreed to live his life on the basis of the ethical and moral precepts that constitute the program of Alcoholics Anonymous. Given this, it is little wonder that lives turn around. Little wonder that the alcoholic begins to emerge from the shattered pieces of his life like a phoenix arising from his ashes. His recovery is tempered by a willingness to accept things as they are—an orientation that is selfless rather than selfish and which is rooted firmly and inextricably in self-honesty with others in all matters.

The new freedom that the Promises talk about is freedom from the tyranny of alcohol and its attendant compulsions and miseries. It is the happiness derived from a sense of self-worth and a sense of being in step with the process of the world. The past is no longer a source of shame because it does not repeat itself continuously in the present, nor is it expected to do so in the future. Because that past provides a kind of map for growth and change, there is no need to shut the door on it. Further, the past can be used as an example to the newcomer to AA and in that use save someone. "I did that and that's how it worked out." "You don't have to repeat it. Learn from my mistakes."

It is the thrust of the first nine Steps to put the individual at peace with himself and at harmony with the world. They relate expectations to daily possibilities. Peace is a necessary byproduct. Serenity, on the other hand, is derived from the spiritual benefits of the program, which naturally accrue to an individual whose life is based on honesty and ethical and moral selflessness in dealing with others. This concept is particularly difficult to grasp but nonetheless true. The more we strive to benefit others and the more we learn to be generous of spirit and heart, the more we seem to gain in the way of spiritual fulfillment and peace. An individual living this life has little or no time for feelings of uselessness or self-pity. We all feel sorry for ourselves from time to time, but we cannot base a life on negativity. All of us are, at one time or another, victims of injustice. All of us have experienced discrimination or the baseless hostility of those who are close to us. Living the first nine Steps of Alcoholics Anonymous, however, and participating in a program that is spiritual at its basis precludes our reacting to these events with negative feelings for any length of time. The program cautions us that we cannot think our way out of such postures but must live our way out of them.

Although the program is principally oriented toward helping people to stop drinking, much more can be derived from living the AA life. As our spirituality increases and our awareness of ourselves acting in concert with the processes of the world that surrounds us increases, we tend to be less self-oriented and more oriented toward the larger whole. In this sense, our entire attitude and outlook on life has changed. This change in worldview and perspective are mandatory for continued sobriety and abstinence from other mind-altering substances. Sobriety is now a way of life. This change comes through the assiduous working of the Twelve Steps.

Those in AA are promised that fear of people and of economic insecurity will leave them. Unreasonable fear of people, objects, and events is a common theme of drunk-a-logues heard in AA meetings everywhere. As the alcohol leaves the body, the world of the alcoholic becomes more predictable and less dominated by fear. Fear of people disappears when the alcoholic no longer feels the need to control them or to hoax them in one way or another. The Promises also say that the alcoholic will lose the fear of economic insecurity. This is not a promise that every recovered alcoholic will become economically successful. It means only that life is based on an acceptance of things as they are. Control is directed toward oneself and excludes externals.

Sober, the alcoholic stands ready to recognize and accept opportunity when it makes itself apparent. The drunken alcoholic, on the other hand, is not available for anything other than more drinking. The Promises are a predictable outcome of involvement in the AA way of life and active, disciplined involvement in the daily regimen of Alcoholics Anonymous. As the Big Book says, "[W]e have ceased fighting anything or anyone—even alcohol."[3] And, finally, "We have entered the world of the Spirit. Our next function is to grow in understanding and effectiveness."[4]

Appendix A

Events in the History of Alcoholics Anonymous

1934   Dr. William D. Silkworth pronounces Bill W. a hopeless alcoholic.
In August, the Oxford Group sobers up Bill's friend Ebby T.
Ebby visits Bill in November and tells him his story.
Bill has a spiritual experience in Towns Hospital in December.

1935   In May, Dr. Bob and Bill meet in Akron, Ohio.
Dr. Bob has his last drink on June 10. Alcoholics Anonymous is
     founded.

1937   New York AA separates from the Oxford Group.
In November, Dr. Bob and Bill meet in Akron, Ohio, and count
     results. Forty cases sober. First realization of certain success.

1938   John D. Rockefeller Jr. contacted. He gives $5,000 in February but
     refuses to give more, saving AA from professionalism.
In May, the Alcoholic Foundation, a trusteeship, is established.
     Writing of the book *Alcoholics Anonymous* begins.
The Twelve Steps are written in December.

1939   Membership reaches 100.
Alcoholics Anonymous is published. Dr. Fosdick reviews it.
Midwestern AA chapters withdraw from the Oxford Group in the
     summer. AA is fully on its own.
Dr. Bob and Sister Ignatia start work at St. Thomas Hospital in
     Akron in August. They treat 5,000 cases in the next ten years.
Sudden expansion in September in Cleveland proves AA can grow
     to great size.
In December, the first AA group in a mental institution is started at
     Rockland State Hospital in New York.

1940   Religious leaders publicly approve AA, e.g., Father Dowling, Dr.
     Fosdick (forerunners of many).

In February, the first world service office for AA is established on Versey Street in New York. The first AA Clubhouse opens at 334½ West 25th Street, New York.

1941   March *Saturday Evening Post* article causes great national expansion and recognition of AA. Membership jumps from 2,000 to 8,000 by year's end.

1942   First prison AA group is formed in San Quentin, California.

1944   The *AA Grapevine* is established in June.

1945   Dr. Silkworth and Teddy R. begin work at Knickerbocker Hospital in New York.
They treat 10,000 cases in the next ten years.

1946   The Twelve Traditions of AA are first formulated and published.

1949   American Psychiatric Association recognizes AA.

1950   First International Convention is held in Cleveland in July. The Twelve Traditions are adopted by the movement.
Dr. Bob dies in November.

1951   First General Service Conference meets in April, beginning a five-year experimental period and linking AA's trustees with the entire fellowship.
In October, the American Public Health Association gives Lasker Award to AA in San Francisco.

1954   The "Alcoholic Foundation" becomes the General Service Board of AA. The original idea of an all-purpose foundation is abandoned.

1956   Public Information Committee is created to assume charge of public relations, which were previously handled by Bill Wilson.

1957   First overseas General Service Board of AA is created in Great Britain and Ireland. AA membership has reached more than 200,000 people in 7,000 groups in 70 countries and U.S. possessions.

1959   AA Publishing, Inc., becomes AA World Services, Inc.

1960   25th Anniversary Convention is held in July in Long Beach, California.
The book *Avec Les Alcooliques,* by Joseph Kessel, stimulates growth of AA in France and Germany.

1961   Bill exchanges letters with Dr. Carl Jung. Dr. Jung's help of an alcoholic in 1930 is later seen as a first step in the formation of AA.

1962   *Twelve Concepts for World Service,* by Bill Wilson, is published.

1963–67 Rapid growth overseas is accelerated by increased world service activity, such as more advisory correspondence, the establishment of new literature centers, large numbers of new and effective translations, and better inculcation of AA traditions.

1965   30th Anniversary Convention in Toronto, Canada is attended by more than 10,000 in July. The Declaration, later so widely used, is the keynote of this gathering: "I Am Responsible. When anyone, anywhere reaches out for help, I want the hand of AA always to be there. And for that: I am responsible." Gift pocket-sized edition of *Twelve Steps and Twelve Traditions* is released. A color film documentary, in which Bill and Lois Wilson tell the early AA story, is produced for group use only.

1966   The ratio of trustees of the General Service Board is changed to provide for a two-thirds majority of alcoholic members. The AA fellowship thus accepts top responsibility for the future conduct of all its affairs. With this change, the number of regional trustees rises to eight (six from the United States, two from Canada).

1967   *The AA Way of Life* (now titled *As Bill Sees It*), featuring extracts from Bill W.'s writings, is published. The number of AA groups increases to 13,279; overseas groups come to represent about 20 percent of the AA population.

1969   First World Service Meeting is held in October in New York, with delegates from 14 countries. (Biennial meetings are held after 1972.)

1970   35th Anniversary International Convention in Miami Beach, Florida, is attended by 11,000. It is Bill's last public appearance. The keynote is the Declaration of Unity.

1971   Bill Wilson dies on January 24. His name, picture, and story are carried worldwide in public media for the first time. AA groups worldwide hold memorial services for him on February 14.

1973   In April, distribution of the book *Alcoholics Anonymous* reaches the 1 million mark.

1975   40th Anniversary International Convention is held in Denver, Colorado.

1976   Worldwide there are an estimated 1 million members and almost 28,000 groups.

1980   Registrations reach 22,500 as members gather in New Orleans to celebrate "The Joy of Living" at the 45th Anniversary AA International Convention. The book *Dr. Bob and the Good Old-timers,* introduced at the convention, combines biography and a history of AA in the Midwest.

1988   Lois Burnham Wilson dies in October.

Source: Adapted from Alcoholics Anonymous World Services, Inc., *Alcoholics Anonymous Comes of Age* (New York: author, 1983), pp. vii–xi.

Appendix B

How It Works, the Steps, and the Traditions

HOW IT WORKS

"How It Works" is a chapter from the Big Book. What follows is the opening portion, which is read at the beginning of meetings.

Rarely have we seen a person fail who has thoroughly followed our path. Those who do not recover are people who cannot or will not completely give themselves to this simple program, usually men and women who are constitutionally incapable of being honest with themselves. There are such unfortunates. They are not at fault; they seem to have been born that way. They are naturally incapable of grasping and developing a manner of living which demands rigorous honesty. Their chances are less than average. There are those, too, who suffer from grave emotional and mental disorders, but many of them do recover if they have the capacity to be honest.

Our stories disclose in a general way what we used to be like, what happened, and what we are like now. If you have decided you want what we have and are willing to go to any length to get it—then you are ready to take certain steps.

At some of these we balked. We thought we could find an easier, softer way. But we could not. With all the earnestness at our command, we beg of you to be fearless and thorough from the very start. Some of us have tried to hold on to our old ideas and the result was nil until we let go absolutely.

Remember that we deal with alcohol—cunning, baffling, powerful! Without help it is too much for us. But there is One who has all power—that One is God. May you find Him now!

Half measures availed us nothing. We stood at the turning point. We asked His protection and care with complete abandon.

Here are the steps we took, which are suggested as a program of recovery:

1. We admitted we were powerless over alcohol—that our lives had become unmanageable.

2. Came to believe that a Power greater than ourselves could restore us to sanity.

3. Made a decision to turn our will and our lives over to the care of God *as we understood Him.*

4. Made a searching and fearless moral inventory of ourselves.

5. Admitted to God, to ourselves, and to another human being the exact nature of our wrongs.

6. Were entirely ready to have God remove all these defects of character.

7. Humbly asked Him to remove our shortcomings.

8. Made a list of all persons we had harmed, and became willing to make amends to them all.

9. Made direct amends to such people wherever possible, except when to do so would injure them or others.

10. Continued to take personal inventory and when we were wrong promptly admitted it.

11. Sought through prayer and meditation to improve our conscious contact with God *as we understood Him,* praying only for knowledge of His will for us and the power to carry that out.

12. Having had a spiritual awakening as the result of these steps, we tried to carry this message to alcoholics, and to practice these principles in all our affairs.

Source: Alcoholics Anonymous World Services, Inc., *Alcoholics Anonymous,* 4th ed., (New York: author, 2001), pp. 58–60. Reprinted with permission.

THE TWELVE TRADITIONS

"The Twelve Traditions," also read at meeting openings, is found, in both its short and long forms, at the end of the Big Book. The short form, which follows, is the one normally used.

1. Our common welfare should come first; personal recovery depends upon AA unity.

2. For our group purpose there is but one ultimate authority—a loving God as He may express Himself in our group conscience. Our leaders are but trusted servants; they do not govern.

3. The only requirement for AA membership is a desire to stop drinking.

4. Each group should be autonomous except in matters affecting other groups or AA as a whole.

5. Each group has but one primary purpose—to carry its message to the alcoholic who still suffers.

6. An AA group ought never endorse, finance or lend the AA name to any related facility or outside enterprise, lest problems of money, property and prestige divert us from our primary purpose.

7. Every AA group ought to be fully self-supporting, declining outside contributions.

8. Alcoholics Anonymous should remain forever nonprofessional, but our service centers may employ special workers.

9. AA, as such, ought never be organized; but we may create service boards or committees directly responsible to those they serve.

10. Alcoholics Anonymous has no opinion on outside issues; hence the AA name ought never to be drawn into public controversy.

11. Our public relations policy is based on attraction rather than promotion; we need always maintain personal anonymity at the level of press, radio and films.

12. Anonymity is the spiritual foundation of all our Traditions, ever reminding us to place principles before personalities.

Source: Alcoholics Anonymous World Services, Inc., *Alcoholics Anonymous*, 4th ed., (New York: author, 2001), p. 562. Reprinted with permission.

Notes

Chapter 1. Alcoholics Anonymous

1. Alcoholics Anonymous World Services, Inc., *Dr. Bob and the Good Oldtimers* (New York: author, 1980), p. 55.

2. Ibid., p. 55. See also Nan Robertson, *Getting Better: Inside Alcoholics Anonymous* (New York: William Morrow & Co., 1988), pp. 60–67.

3. Alcoholics Anonymous World Services, Inc., *Alcoholics Anonymous Comes of Age* (New York: author, 2002), p. 59.

4. Ibid., p. 63.

5. Ibid.

6. Edgar Nace, *The Treatment of Alcoholism* (New York: Brunner/Mazel, 1987), p. 239.

7. Alcoholics Anonymous World Services, Inc., *Alcoholics Anonymous Comes of Age,* p. 124.

8. Alcoholics Anonymous World Services, Inc., *Pass It On: The Story of Bill Wilson and How the Message Reached the World* (New York: author, 1984), pp. 124–25.

9. Ibid., p. 139.

10. Ibid., p. 143.

11. Alcoholics Anonymous World Services, Inc., *Alcoholics Anonymous Comes of Age,* p. 161.

12. Alcoholics Anonymous World Services, Inc., *Pass It On,* p. 171.

13. Ibid., p. 172.

14. Ibid., p. 178.

15. Ibid., p. 198.

16. Ibid., p. 204.

17. Alcoholics Anonymous World Services, Inc., *Alcoholics Anonymous Comes of Age,* p. 103.

18. Ibid., p. 105.

19. Alcoholics Anonymous World Services, Inc., *Alcoholics Anonymous,* 4th ed. (New York: author, 2001), p. 84.

Chapter 2. A Matter of Definition

1. Enoch Gordis, "Improving the Old, Embracing the New: Implications for Alcohol Research for Future Practice," *Social Work in Health Care* 33, no. 1 (2001): 17–41.

2. Ibid., p. 19.

3. E. Mansell Pattison and Edward Kaufman, eds., *Encyclopedic Handbook of Alcoholism* (New York: Gardner Press, 1982), pp. 5–6.

4. American Psychiatric Association, *Diagnostic and Statistical Manual of Mental Disorders DSM-IV-TR* (Washington, D.C.: author, 2000), p. 197.

5. Ibid., 199.

6. World Health Organization, *ICD-10*, Chapter 5, Mental and Behavioural Disorders Due to Psychoactive Substance Use, F10–F19, available at www.who.int/classifications/apps/icd/icd10online/ (accessed February 13, 2007).

7. Ibid.

8. Pattison and Kaufman, *Encyclopedic Handbook of Alcoholism*, p. 9.

9. Ibid.

10. Ibid., p. 10.

11. Ibid., p. 609.

12. E. M. Jellinek, *The Disease Concept of Alcoholism* (New Haven: Hillhouse Press, 1960).

13. E. M. Jellinek, "Phases in the Drinking History of Alcoholics: Analysis of a Survey Conducted by the Official Organ of Alcoholics Anonymous," *Quarterly Journal of Studies on Alcohol,* 7 (1946): 1–88.

14. E. M. Jellinek, "Phases of Alcohol Addiction," *Quarterly Journal of Studies on Alcohol* 13 (1952): 673–84.

15. Pattison and Kaufman, *Encyclopedic Handbook of Alcoholism,* p. 213.

16. Ibid., p.14.

17. Ibid., p. 22.

18. Paul R. McHugh and Phillip R. Slavney, *The Perspectives of Psychiatry,* 2d ed., (Baltimore: Johns Hopkins University Press, 1998), p. 45.

19. Ibid., p. 53.

20. Edgar Nace, *The Treatment of Alcoholism* (New York: Brunner Mazel, 1987), p. 63.

21. Ibid., p. 66.

22. Ibid., p. 68.

23. Gordis, "Improving the Old."

24. Ibid., p. 19.

25. Ibid., p. 29.

26. Ibid.

27. Ibid., p. 34.

28. Philip R. Reilly, *Is It in Your Genes? The Influence of Genes on Common Disorders and Diseases that Affect You and Your Family* (Cold Spring Harbor, N.Y.: Cold Spring Harbor Laboratory Press, 2004), p. 234.

29. Ibid., p. 235.

30. Alcoholics Anonymous World Services, Inc., *Pass It On: The Story of Bill Wilson and How the AA Message Reached the World* (New York: author, 1984), p. 84.

31. Ibid., p. 102.

32. In the folk wisdom of AA, particular ethnic stocks are defined as producing more alcoholics than others. For example, it is commonly held that the Irish statistically produce more alcoholics than other definable national or ethnic groups. In AA there is a slang expression that translates CIA into Catholic, Irish, and Alcoholic. Curiously, although epidemiologically Scandinavians and Germans are frequently cited as having high incidences of alcoholism, they are not designated as such in AA. Environmental issues receive much less interest in AA meetings than they do in the literature. The common understanding is that differences in reported rates of alcoholism among the social classes are the result of

difficulties in reporting or the ability of middle- and upper-class alcoholics to hide their alcoholism rather than reflecting the influence of culture on the incidence of alcoholism. In AA circles, one hears the expression "From Yale to jail, we're all united by a common affliction: alcoholism." The folklore of AA as well as its written literature recognizes the heterogeneity of the population of both AA and the universe of alcoholics.

33. World Health Organization, *ICD-10,* F10–F19.

Chapter 3. Alcohol and the Alcoholic

1. Although the "20 Questions" are identified with AA, they originated as "Hopkins Twenty Questions" and were developed by Wallace Mandell, professor emeritus, Bloomberg School of Public Health, the Johns Hopkins University.

2. Alcoholics Anonymous World Services, Inc., *Alcoholics Anonymous Comes of Age* (New York: author, 2002), pp. 309–10.

Chapter 5. Mending

1. Alcoholics Anonymous World Services, Inc., *Twelve Steps and Twelve Traditions* (New York: author, 1981), p. 21.

2. Ibid., pp. 32–33.
3. Ibid., p. 35.
4. Ibid., p. 41.
5. Ibid., p. 54.
6. Ibid., p. 55.
7. Ibid., p. 68.
8. Ibid., p. 70.
9. Ibid., p. 75.
10. Ibid., p. 76.
11. Ibid., p. 83.
12. Narcotics Anonymous World Services, Inc., *It Works—How and Why: The Twelve Steps and Twelve Traditions of Narcotics Anonymous* (Chatsworth, Calif.: author, 1993), p. 89.
13. Ibid., p. 95.
14. Alcoholics Anonymous World Services, Inc., *Alcoholics Anonymous,* 4th ed. (New York: author, 2001), pp. 83–84.
15. Ibid., p. 84.
16. Ibid.
17. Alcoholics Anonymous World Services, Inc., *Twelve Steps and Twelve Traditions,* p. 88.
18. Ibid., p. 92.

Chapter 7. The Alcoholic and the Family

1. Lois Wilson, *Lois Remembers* (New York: Al-Anon Family Group Headquarters, Inc., 1979). See also Al-Anon Family Group Headquarters, *First Steps: The Initial History of Al-Anon* (New York: author, 1986).

2. J. Albion, "Support Systems Dynamics of Al-Anon and Alateen," in E. Mansell Pattison and Edward Kaufman, eds., *Encyclopedic Handbook of Alcoholism* (New York: Gardner Press, 1982), p. 993.

Chapter 8. The Road to a Life Well Lived

1. Alcoholics Anonymous World Services, Inc., *Alcoholics Anonymous,* 4th ed. (New York: author, 2001), pp. 83–84.

2. Ibid., p. 83.

3. Ibid., p. 84.

4. Ibid.

References

Al-Anon Family Group Headquarters. *First Steps: The Initial History of Al-Anon.* New York: author, 1986.

Albion, J. "Support Systems Dynamics of Al-Anon and Alateen." In E. Mansell Pattison and Edward Kaufman (Eds.), *Encyclopedic Handbook of Alcoholism,* p. 993. New York: Gardner Press, 1982.

Alcoholics Anonymous World Services, Inc. *Alcoholics Anonymous Comes of Age.* New York: author, 2002.

———. *Alcoholics Anonymous.* 4th ed. New York: author, 2001.

———. *Dr. Bob and the Good Oldtimers.* New York: author, 1980.

———. *Pass It On: The Story of Bill Wilson and How the AA Message Reached the World.* New York: author, 1984.

———. *Twelve Steps and Twelve Traditions.* New York: author, 1981.

American Psychiatric Association. *Diagnostic and Statistical Manual of Mental Disorders DSM-IV-TR.* Washington, D.C.: author, 2000.

Gordis, Enoch. "Improving the Old, Embracing the New: Implications for Alcohol Research for Future Practice." *Social Work in Health Care* 33, no. 1 (2001): 17–41.

Jellinek, E. M. "Phases in the Drinking History of Alcoholics: Analysis of a Survey Conducted by the Official Organ of Alcoholics Anonymous." *Quarterly Journal of Studies on Alcohol* 7 (1946): 1–88.

———. "Phases of Alcohol Addiction." *Quarterly Journal of Studies on Alcohol* 13 (1952): 673–84.

———. *The Disease Concept of Alcoholism.* New Haven, Conn.: Hillhouse Press, 1960.

McHugh, Paul R., and Phillip R. Slavney. *The Perspectives of Psychiatry.* 2d ed. Baltimore: Johns Hopkins University Press, 1998.

Nace, Edgar. *The Treatment of Alcoholism.* New York: Brunner/Mazel Publishers, 1987.

Narcotics Anonymous World Services, Inc. *It Works—How and Why: The Twelve Steps and Twelve Traditions of Narcotics Anonymous.* Chatsworth, Calif.: author, 1993.

———. "Who, What, How, and Why." Reprinted from the White Booklet, *Narcotics Anonymous.* Chatsworth, Calif.: author, 1986.

Pattison, E. Mansell, and Edward Kaufman, eds. *Encyclopedic Handbook of Alcoholism.* New York: Gardner Press, 1982.

Reilly, Philip R. *Is It in Your Genes? The Influence of Genes on Common Disorders and Diseases that Affect You and Your Family.* Cold Spring Harbor, N.Y.: Cold Spring Harbor Laboratory Press, 2004.

Robertson, Nan. *Getting Better: Inside Alcoholics Anonymous.* New York: William Morrow & Co., 1988.

Wilson, Lois. *Lois Remembers.* New York: Al-Anon Family Group Headquarters, Inc., 1979.

World Health Organization. *International Statistical Classification of Diseases and Problems.* 10th Revision. 2006. Chapter V, Mental and Behavioural Disorders Due to Psychoactive Substance Use, F10–F19. On-line manual. Available at www.who.int/classifications/apps/icd/icd10online/ (accessed February 13, 2007).

Index

absolutes, rejection of, 11
agnostics, and prayer, 140
Al-Anon, 62, 64, 155–160
Alateen, 157
alcohol: compared with drug addiction, 134–136; influence on personality, 55; reasons for initial use, 47; social definition, 26
alcoholics: attitude toward family and sobriety, 161; child, 171; obsession of, and compulsive nature, 39; personality type, 53; social class and drinking patterns, 72; social fit, 70; stereotypes, 66
Alcoholics Anonymous: alcoholism defined (physical, mental, spiritual), 45; the Big Book (1939), 13–14; break with Oxford Group, 10; history highlights, 189–192; philosophical foundations, 99; prologue, at start of meetings, 14; traditions, 10
alcoholism: age at first drink, 37; compulsion to drink, 68; as disease, 33; early stages, 50; family disease, 148; functional definition, 42; genetic role, 37; later stages, 54; loss of "fit" in the culture, 68; psychological impact, 52–53; spirituality, 61; twin studies, 36
Amends Step, 114
anonymity, origins of, 9

Big Book, 13–14
binge drinker, 52
bottom, perspectives, 71, 76
Buchman, Frank, 4; support of Hitler, 11

change, breaking patterns, 85
children of alcoholic parents, 172–174
codependence, 80
compulsion to drink, 49, 179
court slips and boundary issues, 136
creativity and alcohol, 180

denial, 58; and enabling, 148
Diagnostic and Statistical Manual of Mental Diseases. See DSM IV-TR

disease of alcoholism, common currency in AA, 39
disease model, 33–34
drinking after sobriety, progressive nature of alcoholism, 41
drugs and alcohol, 134
drunk-a-logue, 4; alcoholic's story, 14
DSM IV-TR, definitions, criteria for alcohol dependence, abuse, 26
dual addiction, 134

Ebby T., 4; religious experience, 6
emotional growth stunted by alcoholism, 62
enabling, 148–149; consequences of, 150; family, 79; spouses, 154

families, socialization and control, 174
family, perceptions of alcoholism's impact, 166
fellowship, discussion of, 20

getting sober, process of, 80
Gordis, Enoch: alcohol research, 35; definition of alcoholism, 36; scope of alcohol/drug problems in the U.S., 25

healing, abstinence, 50
higher power, 91
honest program, 128
How It Works, the Steps, and the Traditions, 193–194

ICD-10, definition of alcoholism, 28
insanity, AA's definition of, 95
International Classification of Diseases. See ICD-10
interpersonal relationships and recovery, 150
interventions, 72

James, William, influence on AA philosophy, 8
Jellinek, E. M., 30
Jellinek's Curve, 30–32

maintenance drinking, 29
Maintenance Steps, 119
McHugh, Paul R., & Phillip R. Slavney, on def-
    inition of disease, 33
meetings, 14; based on fellowship, 17; formed
    by any group of people for sobriety, 181;
    membership runs, 17; purpose of and reac-
    tions to, 23; types, 16; why and how, 82
Moral Re-Armament Group, 5
multivariate syndrome, 32

Nace, Edgar, on multivariate syndrome, dis-
    ease as applicable term, 34
ninety meetings in ninety days, 82

obsession to drink, 58
Oxford Group, 4–5; AA break from, 10–11; ab-
    solutes, the C's, procedures, 5; publicity and
    public identity, 9

Pattison, E. Mansell, & Edward Kaufman, on
    adverse consequences of alcoholism, 28
prayer: importance of content, 139; and resent-
    ments, 138; sobriety, 137
program, importance of involvement in, 146
progressive disease, alcoholism as, 40
Promises, The, 118, 182; consequence of behav-
    ior, 184

rationalization and denial, 77–78
Reilly, Philip R., on relationship of genes to al-
    coholism, 38
repair, order of (physical, mental, spiritual), 92

sharing, discussion of, 21
Siberling, Henrietta, 7
Silkworth, Dr. William D., and definitions of
    alcoholism: AA, 38; obsession-allergy, 10
slips, return to drinking, 16; consequences of,
    81
slogans, 18–19, 141–145
Smith, Dr. Robert, 8; first meeting, 7

sobriety: concerns of everyday, 132; functional
    definition, 79
social drinker, 30
social role and drinking, 154
spiritual awakening, 123
spiritual axiom, 145
spirituality and alcoholism, 61; and sobriety,
    178
spiritual life, in the culture, 183
sponsor: choice and role, 127; obtaining, 125;
    reciprocal nature of, 129
Step One, 93, 102
Step Two, 93, 105
Step Three, 96, 105
Step Four, 97, 106
Step Five, 97, 106–107
Step Six, 98, 108
Step Seven, 98, 108–110
Step Eight, 98, 113
Step Nine, 98, 115
Step Ten, 119–123
Step Eleven, 119–123
Step Twelve, 119–123
Steps, 87; list of, 194; secular view, 91–99; tradi-
    tional perspective, 99–117
substance abuse criteria, 27

threats to sobriety, 130
Tiebout, Harry M., and early AA, 56–57
Towns Hospital (New York), 6
Twelve and Twelve, The, 105, 193–195; tolerance
    for self and fellows, 122
Twelve Traditions, The, 194–195
Twenty Questions, 53–54

Wilson Bill, & Dr. Robert Smith, in Detroit for
    early program evaluation, 12
Wilson, Bill, 4; begins writing the Big Book in
    1938, 13; last detox, 6; reflections on first
    meeting, 9; split with Oxford Group, 11
Wilson, Lois: founded Al-Anon, 157–158; on
    writing of Steps, 13

Jack H. Hedblom received his Ph.D. in sociology from the State University of New York at Buffalo and his M.S.W. from the University of Maryland. He has held faculty positions at major universities and published in the areas of human sexuality, social deviance, criminology, and methods of social research. He has co-authored two books and contributed chapters to others in the areas of social policy and penology. He began a private psychotherapy practice after serving as a clinician at the Veterans Administration Hospital in Baltimore. He lives with his wife and two collies in the Baltimore area.